The Rainbow

Words of Inspiration, Faith and Hope

By

Ferna Lary Mills

ISBN: 978-1-4033-0420-9 (sc)
ISBN: 978-1-4033-0419-3 (e)

This book is printed on acid free paper.

1stBooks - rev. 01/22/03

THE RAINBOW

We cannot grasp it in our hand.
It's beginning and end we cannot see.
That brilliant multicolored band
He placed in the sky for you and me.

It's His promise of a brighter day
long after this storm has passed,
to remind us in a special way
that these sorrows will not last.

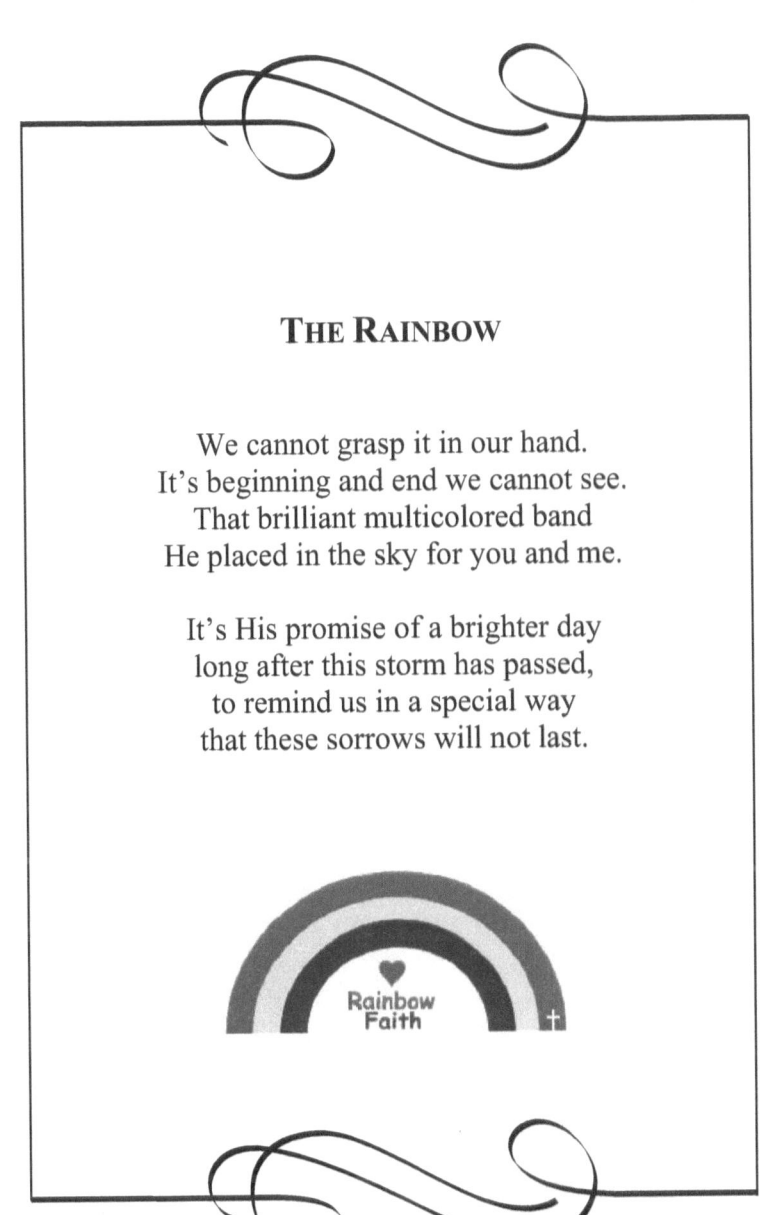

Be merciful to me, O Lord, for I am in distress;
My eyes grow weak with worry, my soul and my body with grief.
Psalms 31:9

DEDICATION

To Wayne and Sara,
my two real-life heroes.

In Memory

In loving memory of my parents, Marian and Bill. They weren't perfect, but they were wonderful parents. Poppa was my strength and my anchor. Mother was my mentor and my life-long best friend. They left behind many wonderful memories, a strong belief in the capacity of the human spirit, and a solid faith in God above.

Marian Irene O'Dell Rodgers
November 28, 1933 - April 30, 1999

Billie Wayne Lary
November 13, 1926 - February 14, 2000

TABLE OF CONTENTS

"The Lord bless you and keep you;
the Lord make his face shine upon you
and be gracious to you;
the Lord turn his face toward you
and give you peace."
Numbers 6:24-26

GOOD GRIEF!
THERE IS LIFE AFTER DEATH

Oh, please tell me Lord, how I can go on?
My soul has been crushed into fine silt,
sifting through the mangled pieces of my broken heart.
What morsel of strength is left inside this empty shell?
How can my life possibly continue on?
How can I dream that I will ever feel, breathe, or smile again?
Am I lost forever in this dark tunnel of anguish,
destined to wander forever aimlessly
with no hope of escaping this wretched pain in my soul?

Life is so full of wonder. Each spirit so unique.

Into each and every heart springs forth joy, hope, faith, trust, and elation caused by the multitude of events that happen throughout a natural lifetime.

A wondrous birth.
>A child's wedding.
>>A faithful love.
>>>Anniversaries.
>>>>Grandchildren.

Each individual is given varying measures of each, based on individual circumstances in our lives. That's what makes us so unique. No two people share the exact same joys in their life, in the exact same quantities, but we each have our own portion of joy.

What draws us together into a bond of "sameness" is that at some point along the way, the strength of our hearts is tested with despair, grief, and dark, painful agony. For no matter how our lives begin, or whose life happens to touch ours during a lifetime, at some point every one of us will have to face a death of someone very dear to us. In this sameness, none of us are immune.

For millions of us, the agony of grief did not simply begin when our loved one died. It began weeks, months, or maybe even years prior to that death event as we watched someone very dear to us lose their health. Who can begin to describe the pain in our hearts as we watched them deteriorate before our very eyes day by day? As we cared for them, feeling so helpless? As we mourned for them, long before their passing?

A sudden death in a family is no easier to bear. The shock, the disbelief, and the outrage are in some ways even greater. Our souls cry out in pain when a loved one is wrenched from our life. Here one day. Gone the next. We sit with an empty heart and empty hands and tears wash down our face, shocked by the horrible finality of it. Even when our loved ones struggled with death for so long before letting go and we thought we were so ready, so prepared, we find we were neither.

Death is a part of life. No one is immune to the myriad of emotions that accompanies grief. Whether we have lost our spouse, mother or father, a brother or sister, a friend, a neighbor, co-worker or an old faithful pet, the void is there. The pain and shock are there. The anger and the fear. The despair. The helplessness and the hopelessness strike each of us as we venture reluctantly forward along this journey called Grief.

Left behind, we struggle to find our way in a world suddenly void of all the familiar landmarks. The realities of our life instantly become surreal. Life as we knew it every day of our being up to this point, suddenly no longer exists. The world grows a hundred fold almost overnight. We feel isolated and alone in a strange land once *Death* has struck in our homes and in our hearts.

The mystery is complicated by the fact that the sun still comes up in the morning whether we want it to or not. The birds still sing. The clock still chimes at every hour on the hour. The pages of the calendar still flip by one by one, albeit maybe slower than before. But the old saying still holds true: "Life DOES go on."

How long will the pain last? That depends. How long will you continue to love them? You will always love them and cherish their memories, so the pain will never completely go away. But it will fade in time to a tolerable level. One day peace will be restored to your soul.

The poems, essays and miscellany within the pages of this book were written from the bottom of my heart, and from my spirit to yours. It's my prayer that they will bring hope to those who are in despair, courage to those feeling the intense vulnerability that comes with grief, and faith to those wandering without direction or purpose.

There is STILL meaning and purpose to your life.
Happy times WILL come again.

May God be with you through this difficult time and may the words written in this book speak to your spirit in a special way.

SONG OF MY SOUL

the songs are all off key
the words just will not rhyme
the melody means nothing to me
the rhythm is not keeping time

the comfort just isn't there
the grief overshadows all
the spirit cries in despair
the clock slows down to a crawl

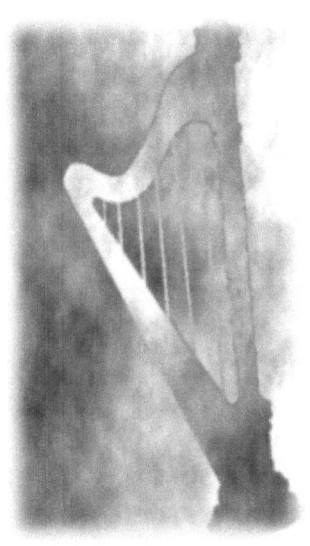

the span of my grief is immense
the heart is engulfed in gloom
the pain in my soul is intense
the song of my soul out of tune

Then you will call, and the Lord will answer;
you will cry for help, and he will say: "Here I am."
Isaiah 58:9

GRIEF IS PERSONAL

Grief is very personal. It's yours and yours alone. No, you aren't the first person to experience grief. But you are the first person to experience YOUR grief. You must deal with it in your own way, in your own time, and on your own terms. Sure, others will have plenty of advice on the things you should do to try to overcome this sudden void in your life; things they think will help you. But the truth is, you must handle it on your own. What worked for them, might work for you. Might not.

You're filled with so many emotions, ranging from despair to anger, and from tears to rage. But how you deal with these emotions is your own personal quest. Someone you loved deeply is never again going to be physically active in your life. Nothing you can do is going to bring them back. That's the aching reality of it all.

Although grief's emotions range across a wide spectrum, everyone will feel each emotion to some degree or another. Some of us hang on to the tears, others get caught up in the rage. Some cannot make themselves feel anything for a long time, allowing the shock to keep them numb and protected while they take solace in it.

There is no magical process to help you get through the pain. No short cuts. Grief hurts. A broken heart or a broken spirit hurts more than broken bones. But there is hope, and having survived this emotional roller coaster, there are a few things I want to share that may help you along the journey to healing.

First, understand that your grief is real, even though everything may have an "unreal" feeling to it. It's not something you are used to, or were prepared for. None of us ever successfully completed SORROW 101. And even though reality bites, acceptance of this reality will be the first major hurdle.

Your life after losing a loved one is vastly different that the life you had while they were still here on this earth. But you must concentrate on the fact that in many ways, your life is still the same. You still live, breathe, need, and feel. Concentrate on the basics at first: food and sleep, even though both may be difficult. As you can, work up to the other things. As bad as it hurts, you are still alive, and there is a reason why. One you will learn in time.

Spend some time alone in your thoughts so you can express your grief without worrying about what others may think. If you want to cry, then cry. If you want to punch something, punch something inanimate - and soft, so you don't hurt yourself. But go ahead. Punch something. No one is watching. You are dealing with your grief in your own way and those hurtful emotions need vented. If you reach a point where you are fighting to hold back the tears, it's time to cry. They need to come out. With each tear that falls, a little grief is washed away.

Take some time out of your life to get a grip on your inner feelings. If you can manage it, you needn't go back to work right away. You don't have to act like nothing in your life has changed. It has! Give yourself time to adjust.

It doesn't take a formal invitation to invite a friend over for coffee. Nor does it take a formal prayer to invite God, your closest friend, to visit with you as you express your feelings. Just pray. He will listen and He wants to carry your burdens. He is only waiting for you to ask. Your faith may be tested during grief as you struggle with so many unanswered questions: why? why now? what now? But remember that only God has all the answers, so it makes perfect sense to stay as close to Him as possible.

Remember your loved one in a special way that means something special to you through a memorial of some kind. It doesn't have to be huge. It doesn't even have to be public. It can be a simple letter to your loved one, a photograph displayed in a special place on the mantle, a rose in a special vase, a poem. Be as creative as you feel.

Eventually, there will come a time that you will realize you can't be an island. You were not meant to walk alone in this world. Sometimes, the hardest part is reaching out to others. Let people into your life. A good friend isn't hard to find if you reach out to them. Let them share your burden, be a shoulder to lean on, and something in your life with some solid stability. Burdens are heavy and are much easier to carry when you don't try to carry them alone.

When you're strong enough, continue reaching out and help others in some way. Even though this may seem impossible to you right now, it will strengthen you as you begin to focus on things outside of yourself. Most importantly, continue to spend time in prayer. God will help mend your broken heart and lead and guide you to find that purpose left in your life. He still has great joys planned for you. Read the scriptures and seek that "peace that surpasses understanding."

Remember this, as dark as it seems right now, there will come a day when your grief will no longer overpower you. You will rise with a strength you didn't even know you possessed, and you WILL live again. In time, you will even smile again.

PRESCRIPTION FOR GRIEF

In a small glass, add
one ounce of hope,
two scoops of courage,
a cup of faith,
and a large portion of prayer.

Mix thoroughly and wash down
with a bucket of tears
and a generous portion of time.

Take as often as needed.

If symptoms persist,
take an extra portion of prayer
and call a friend in the morning.

A POETIC JOURNEY THROUGH GRIEF

The following is a unique trilogy of poems, each one being complete within itself, but part of a "whole" in describing the grief process. Although time doesn't heal all wounds, it does give you the space you need to conduct your own healing.

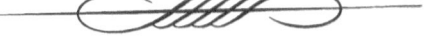

WHEN MY GRIEF WAS NEW

Bury my head in the sand
'til my heart no longer cries,
for there's no pain like the pain you feel
when a loved one dies.

Bury my heart in the ground
'til the very last moment in time,
for there's nothing left inside me to give,
no poems left in me to rhyme.

Bury my soul in the sea
'til the waters turn into clay,
for there's nothing left to hope for now
that my love has gone away.

Bury my hopes and dreams
and my laughter and smiles, too,
for there's no one left on the face of this earth
that cares if I ever do.

Bury me last but not least
in the grave by my loved one's side,
and let peace return to this lonesome beast
since my loved one died.

The second poem in the trilogy:
A Poetic Journey Through Grief

ALONG GRIEF'S JOURNEY

I hear little children laughing
and the sound brings my soul such pain.
Yet, I know in my heart that life goes on
and I must learn to live again.

Some days I stay so busy
I don't even realize you're gone.
Then there are all of those other days when
I feel like I can't go on.

Sometimes I think I dreamed you…
that you never existed for real.
You've been gone so long and I'm just not strong
for my life has become unreal.

They tell me it's time to let go
and build a new life without you.
But the builder is weak and I can't even speak
and I don't know what else to do.

How long will this pain last, Lord?
How many tears have I already cried?
It seems like forever since my world fell apart
when my loved one died.

The final poem in the trilogy:
A POETIC JOURNEY THROUGH GRIEF

PEACE IN MY SOUL

It was such an awesome day
and I stopped to stare up at the sky.
My heart skipped a beat as I heard you speak
when you asked the angel, "Why?"

"I wrote 'I love you' in the sky
as big and as plain as can be.
How can she stand down there and look up here
and still not be able to see?"

The clouds were broken and thin,
and swirled randomly through the air.
I searched and strained at all that remained
of the swirls of white still there.

The angel's voice was soft and low
as I smiled and raised my brow,
and I heard her say in the sweetest way
"She's starting to see it now."

There's a bittersweet peace in my soul
and a sense of awesome pride
knowing you're up there writing words in the air,
and our love has never died.

THE BUTTERFLY

I believe everything was created for a reason. That God, in His infinite wisdom, knew exactly what He was doing during creation, and that nothing was an accident or a mistake. For to believe otherwise, would be to believe in a flawed God.

I believe the giraffe was created intentionally with a long neck to bring us joy. Who can watch without smiling as it stretches it neck into the tree tops for its food, or dips its head down towards a pool of water to drink? I believe the giraffe is symbolic of God's special love for the unique. Such love, that after creating the giraffe, He decided to create each of us the same in some ways, and yet He made each one of us quite unique in many ways.

I believe the fly was created as an annoyance to us in the hot summertime, solely to make us grateful for its absence. Sometimes irritants in our lives are necessary to help us appreciate the good things.

I believe the orangutan was created to make us laugh, the porcupine to make us wary, the zebra to make us wonder, and the butterfly to keep us in awe of God.

Now, think for a moment about the butterfly. I don't believe God ever created a butterfly. Nor has a butterfly ever been "born" to butterfly parents. God created the caterpillar, but He took it one step farther and created it to BECOME a butterfly. He created the process and the means for it to become what He ultimately intends for it to be. Does the caterpillar ever realizes it's purpose? Does it know it's going to become a butterfly? Or does it live it's entire life believing it's only a caterpillar?

It inches along throughout its life, overcoming one obstacle after another. Its only joy is finding food it can devour, and surviving attacks from larger members of the food chain. But it continues on towards God's purpose and design for it: to become a butterfly.

When its life as a caterpillar has been fulfilled, its useless body wraps itself into a cocoon and seals itself to hide the creature it once was.

The caterpillar is no more. Is it dead? No. It just isn't a caterpillar any longer. For once the cocoon opens, a new creature emerges, more beautiful than anything the caterpillar could ever imagine itself to be, even if it had the knowledge that it was going to change appearance. It extends its magnificent wings and flies off into the Heavens as a beautiful butterfly.

If you think people cannot change their appearance, then think of when you were a baby. Now look into the mirror. You are not that same child. You are a new creature, an adult. You are still basically the same on the inside, only drastically different on the outside. How many times over the years have you shed the old and donned the new? Your photographs will show you the evidence.

As the caterpillar changes, so we shall change. When life on earth is ended, we wrap the worn and weary body in a casket and mourn for our loss. But wait! Have they truly died? Like the caterpillar, they have shed the old body. They will emerge new again and rise from their cocoon, more beautiful than ever imagined as they rise towards the Heavens to meet a loving God.

Death is not the end of life. It's only the end of the shell that houses that wonderful life you hold inside. It's not the end of life any more than a cocoon is the end of the life of the caterpillar. It's a new beginning!

We are born into our parents arms from a darkened womb into the light of the world. On the day we accept Christ into our hearts as our own personal Saviour, we are born again into our Father's grace from a world darkened by sin, to dwell in the light of His love. When our final days on this earth are ended, we shed our mortal bodies and we are born finally into the Father's arms as we enter into the Heavenly light of eternity. Three births, each moving us toward becoming the creature He created us to become!

Jesus said, "I tell you the truth, no one can see the
kingdom of God unless he is born again."
John 3:3

It's About Time

Twenty-four hours in a day, seven days in a week, fifty-two weeks in a year. Breakfast time, lunch time, nap time, dinner time, bed time. Measurable time. A lifetime.

Time was created to help us determine where we in the grand scheme of things. It's time for growing up. It's time to save for the future. It's time to eat. It's time to sleep. There is a time for everything. Time to reap. Time to sew. There's a time to laugh, a time to cry, a time to grieve, a time to hang on, and a time to let go.

A loved one dies, and we hear, "It was there time."

I always want to ask, "Oh, according to WHO?" There is never a right time. Death always comes at the wrong time. But what really is this "time" I keep referring to?

All of this time is from a human perspective. I know you are wrinkling your brow at that. But our mechanical clocks and our calendars were created by man, not God. Can you, with all your worries and woes, add one single moment in time to your life's clock? Can you add some extra hours to a day for doing other things you've put off for so long? I think not. So for just a moment, I'm going to ask you to think about God's perspective of time.

God is eternal. He was in the beginning and has been for all time. There has never been a time that God was not. Oh, it's so difficult for a finite mind to understand an infinite God. But because of his infinite existence, our measurements of time mean nothing to Him. When He looks at you, He sees you in the eternal present! Think about that a moment. What a concept!

He doesn't see you as you are this very moment, as your children, family, or others see you. He sees you from the moment you were conceived in his thoughts until the end of eternity, today being only a minuscule portion of the "you" in all of His plan. From the beginning of time until the end of time, he sees you completely in an instant.

Inside and out. Forever and always. Every aspect of you. He sees your past, your present, and your future all at the same time. No wonder we have so much trouble grasping that concept.

Several years ago, a very dear friend reminded me of something I knew but had never actually realized or put into so many words. I was having some problems in parenting and beginning to feel like I had failed. My child was nearing the age of eighteen and still so very far from becoming an adult. I wasn't finished as a parent yet, and I felt like time was quickly running out.

My friend said, "Remember, you are not a parent for just eighteen short years. You are a parent forever. There is no deadline."

I knew that. But, suddenly I realized that youth is such a short amount of time compared to an entire lifetime. And our lifetime is so short compared to all of eternity. We often get bogged down in our day to day lives thinking this is all there is and there's so much to do before we are finished. Comparing our short lifetime on this earth to all of eternity has a way of putting everything back in perspective.

Time on earth is so very short. God's time is infinite. Never ending. So is His love, and both His love and His timing are always perfect. Not until the day we can see things from His perspective, will we ever fully comprehend His timing, nor His perfect love.

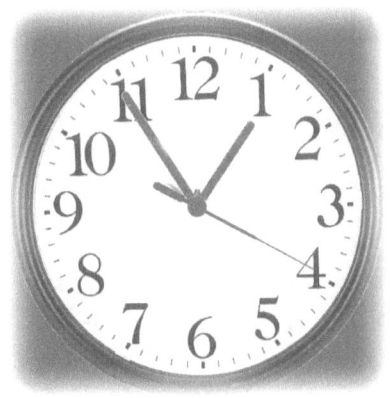

There is a time for everything, and a season for every purpose under Heaven: a time to be born and a time to die.
Ecclesiastes 3: 1, 5

Ferna Lary Mills

GOD'S ONE MISTAKE

With these few lines I wish to convey
the thoughts that fill my mind.
Thoughts of a wonderful yesterday
of a woman who was an Angel
before her time.

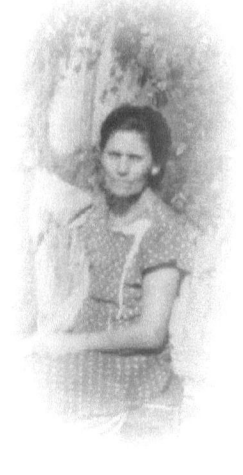

When I was a baby, premature and weak,
and unable to lift even my head,
two pounds of bones she held to her cheek.
She loved me and caressed me.
She made sure I was fed.

And then as I grew to be a man
along with the other nine,
this Angel walked with me and held my hand.
She led me. She guided me.
She shaped my mind.

Then her time came and she was called away
to live with her God in the sky.
She never complained.
She thought of others always.
With a world so full of bad,
why must the wonderful die?

God made one mistake in his overall plan
when He gave unto man his birth.
Angels were to wear halos in the
Promised Land.
Mother wore hers here on earth.

(This poem was written by my father, Billie Wayne Lary, after the death of his mother, Maggie, in 1970. It's included here in their memory.)

14

I WONDER

I wonder how many grains of sand are in an hour glass. Has anyone ever counted them? Does every hour glass contain the same number of grains? Does someone somewhere have a job title of "Sand Grain Counter"? I wonder about all sorts of mundane things these days because it keeps my mind off my grief.

I wonder if I will ever get beyond the pain. How many grains of sand must pass through the hour glass before the hurting stops? How long will the pain last?

I wonder why I never took the time to stop and appreciate the little things I had until they were taken from me. Was I really that busy? What did I have in my life that was more important?

There are so many things I miss that I took for granted while she was alive. What I wouldn't give to bring one minute of them back. It's strange how the things that annoyed me before, I now miss the most.

I miss hearing her shoes shuffling as she moved across the room, never fully lifting her feet from the floor.

I miss listening to her talk non-stop about something she thought was so important, but I did not.

I miss the little things like how she was always waiting with a glass of ice cold tea for me when I finished mowing the grass. I can still taste her iced tea. I remember how refreshingly sweet it tasted on a hot summer day as the sweat ran down my back. I get angry because I can never make a glass of tea taste that good ever again.

I miss how she could understand me better than anyone else on this planet. She knew me inside and out. So many things were communicated between us with just a glance or a smile.

I miss having someone who has a history with me, so memories can be shared without reciting the entire event. Just a basic comment and we could both burst into laughter just from the memory. She was the witness to my own life and history. My note taker. She made my existence on this planet seem real.

I miss her hugs and the shampoo smell of her hair.

I miss her laughter. That twinkle she would get in her eyes. She could never laugh without tears. She called them her tears of joy. Sometimes she could find humor in the simplest things. It's almost as if it was her sole duty in life to find things that would make me laugh. We would laugh so long that we forgot what it was that got us started. Our sides would ache but we would still laugh anyway. Then one glance at one another and we would take off again in fits of laughter. I miss the joy she created in our home.

Grief hurts. It makes my throat dry, my eyes burn, my stomach ache and hurts my heart. I am constantly amazed that the broken heart inside my chest still keeps on beating. It feels like there's a hole in my heart and all my hopes and dreams fell out of it leaving a giant void I'll never be able to fill. I search constantly trying to find something to fill this empty space and nothing seems to work. I struggle to avoid filling it with guilt, anger or despair.

Grief is a result of wanting her so badly and knowing I can no longer have her with me. Absolute grief comes from wanting her absolutely. My head knows she is gone, but my heart says I'm not ready to let her go yet. These two pieces of me need to have a serious discussion with each other, for I know that only when they come to an agreement and allow me to be honest about my loss will true healing ever begin.

Distractions keep my mind off my grief during the day, but the nighttime's are the worst. Sudden waves of grief seemingly come out of nowhere when I least expect it. A word. A memory. It all comes flooding over me. I can only try to cope one moment at a time. And sometimes that seems impossible.

I'm still in shock over the finality of her death. The permanency of it. And I wonder if people who commit suicide ever really completely understand death's finality. I don't believe they do. Death doesn't abide by any of our terms. It's final. No reprieves, no parole, no second chances. Once the curtain is down, the show is over. No credits given. No bylines. No awards. If not for the memories in the minds of the audience, it's as if it never played.

My torment mounts as I realize how much love I still have left inside of me, with no one left to take it. Then I realize with a sense of surprise that the love inside of me didn't die with her. It's still here. Waiting.

My children still need tons of this love. They are still here, even though for a while I could see nothing but my own grief. Yes, I have good friends and other family members close by. They are all takers and givers of this love. I still have my faith. And no love is greater than His.

I still have to give love to myself if I want to continue to exist. No matter how broken my heart may be, I am still capable of love. If I cannot eat or sleep, or concentrate, or make decisions, or find anything to get my mind off my grief for a little while, I can still love and be loved.

Grief causes me to find the courage within myself to reach out to others who are also hurting. She left more than one of us behind. I'm not the only person in the world she ever connected with, cared for, or touched. I'm not the only one hurting by her absence. In spite of myself, I feel better just being with other people she loved. It reaffirms to me that she truly did exist. It also reminds me that I still exist, too. By keeping the love alive we can also keep ourselves alive.

Life is still worth living. My grief has greatly diminished my expectations of life, but not life itself. There is no measuring stick to measure where I am in my grief, or to show that I'm progressing or lagging behind. But as I continue to love my family and friends, reach out to others, and seek solace in a power higher than myself, I will come through this. Although sometimes I feel so very alone, I realize I cannot make it through this life alone.

I wonder how many sea shells are on the seashore. I wonder if all of the sand on the beach is just ground up sea shells. Is there really any sand on the beach at all? I wonder if the sand in the hour glass is made from ground up sea shells.

LETTER FROM HEAVEN

I felt your soft touch and heard your mournful cry.
You knew I was leaving, but you couldn't grasp "why".
You held onto my hand, your heart heavy with gloom,
As I passed from this lifetime and rose up from the room.

It happened so quickly, in the blink of an eye.
My heart was too weak. No strength for "goodbye".
You saw it, I know, how the light drained from my face,
But you missed His great GLORY as it lit up the place.

I yearned so to hold you and say, "It's okay",
But He took my hand and said, "Let's be on our way."
Please don't grieve for me now, love, for I have not died.
He just put out this lamp for my dawn has arrived.

Though I'll miss you intensely, as I know you'll miss me,
He has places to take me, and wondrous things I shall see.
I've been reborn to a place you can't now understand;
A place of Glory, and Peace, nestled in His right hand.

Yet I'll be with you always, only a faint breath away.
My love shall be with you every moment, every day.
And although I don't know yet every step of His plan,
Rest secure in the knowledge that we WILL meet again!

GONE ONLY FROM MY SIGHT

The little toddler curls his tiny fingers and waves just the way his parents taught him. His smile is bright and his eyes sparkle as he sings, "Bye-Bye." It's one of the first things we learn as children. How to say goodbye. Whether it's off to daycare, to school, or to Grandma's house, we wave and smile and sing, "Bye-Bye."

I was so angry when my mother left me. I knew she would never come back and the finality of her leaving made saying "Bye-Bye" impossible. I just couldn't force myself to tell her goodbye this time. Oh, I had told her that so many times over the years with a smile on my face. Off to school, down the aisle when I married, off to a new town in another part of the country with my new family, at the end of a too-short visit, or at the end of a too-long telephone call.

But this time it was different. This time she was leaving, not me. This time it was final. She wouldn't be coming back. Cancer made sure of that.

I watched her frail body give in to her illness and then she left me. Angry tears washed down my face because I new she wasn't coming back. It wasn't fair. I wasn't finished with her yet. I still had too many things to ask her, and too many days I would need her, and yet she still left. Just like that, she was gone from me.

Surely, I thought, there must be someone I can blame. Someone who is responsible for this injustice. I wanted to be mad at her, but it wasn't her fault. She didn't plan on getting cancer. She wanted to get well. She never wanted to die. She never wanted to leave me.

I was so angry that I wasn't able to tell her goodbye. I couldn't make the words come because I knew it was going to be so damned final.

I wanted to be angry at God for taking her too soon. They say God doesn't make mistakes, but I was certain that this time He had. And it was a big one. But while I was trying to aim my anger, I suddenly recalled an event many years earlier in my life. It played out before me as in an old home movie.

My family had moved, which it seemed we did often due to my father's occupation. Mother searched until she finally found a church in our new hometown. It was our first Sunday there.

She dropped me off at the door of my new Sunday School class with a dozen or so other five-year-old little girls. She smiled her Mommy smile and said, "I'll be back, hon. Remember, I'm just out of sight for a little while."

Well, I didn't feel five. I felt more like two. I didn't want her to go away and leave me alone with all those strange children. I didn't know any of them and I wasn't sure I even wanted to. I just wanted the comfort of having her beside me. With her close to me, I could handle anything, even ten dozen strangers. But she left me there anyway, and for what seemed like a gazillion hours, she was gone. I was still crying when she returned and she was sorely surprised that I had reacted so strongly to her leaving.

When we got home she sat down and tenderly spoke these words to me with all the love in her heart and a great big smile on her face: "Remember when I left you this morning? You know something really amazing? I wasn't really gone!"

Those words struck me as a lie. A Sunday lie, which was even worse. Sure she was gone. She left, and was gone. And I was all alone. I had watched the door for forever before she came back to get me. I stared at her with disbelief as she continued.

"I was only out of your sight. I left the room you were in, and I went into another room. But I was still there. Don't you see? I'm never really gone. Just, sometimes I'm out of your sight for awhile."

I remember being so confused. She was so sincere and I could feel the love in her voice. She had sparkles in her eyes as she told me this story. It was like she had been on an adventure.

"Even though I wasn't with you, I carried you in my heart the entire time I was in the other room. I thought about you constantly, and couldn't wait to get back to see you again. You are my shining star. But see, when I got back and saw you still crying, it just broke my heart. Don't you know I'm with you always, even when I'm away for just a little while? I will always love you. Always! Even when I have to be gone from your sight for just a little while."

I don't claim to have all the answers about life and death, or life after death. But I know in my heart that she is now only gone from my sight.

She still carries me with her in her heart, wherever she has gone. For whatever time I have left on this earth, I will carry her in my heart. Someday we will meet again, and the gazillion hours of waiting will be over. I don't want to be caught still crying when we meet again. I don't want to break her heart. I want to look into her eyes and hear her say, "I'm so proud of you, hon."

There's a story about the dying process that uses an analogy of a ship leaving the shore. As the ship moves out into the deep waters it appears to get smaller, but its size actually always remains the same. It only diminishes in our sight. While we stand at the shore and wave goodbye, it disappears from our sight and we cry, "There she goes."

What we cannot see is the distant shore. Others stand alongside the water and cheer as the ship approaches. They shout with abundant joy, "Here she comes!"

Some glorious day I will get to stand on that other shore and share in her great adventure.

I go to prepare a place for you.
And if I go and prepare a place for you, I will come again
and take you to be with me that you may also be where I am.
You know the way to the place where I am going.
John 14:1-4

THE LIGHT

There's a beautiful light in the distance,
yet I see it only at night, in my dreams.
It's impossible to see while I'm awake
and I'm not sure I know what it means.

It's like sunlight on a cold gray morning,
yet it warms from inside the soul
with the warmth of a hot summer sun
melting away the harsh winter cold.

The light? Now I see when I'm near Him,
it grows bright enough to see during the day.
So I'll let Him guide me towards it
and be my strength as He shows me the way.

Lord, be my strength and my guide,
teach me to be strong and to trust in You,
and this light will continue to grow brighter
even in this darkness I must pass through.

When I'm frightened or feeling abandoned,
or feel the darkness closing in around me,
let Your light shine bright in my soul, Lord,
for I know that one day I'll be free.

The light grows brighter and brighter.
The darkness in my soul fades away.
And beside you, Lord, nestled in your love,
Is where I will forever stay.

Then Jesus spoke again to them, saying, "I am the light of the world:
he that follows me shall not walk in darkness
but shall have the light of life."
John 8:12

THE ROSES

It was a bad year for the roses.

March roared in and collapsed my world. My mother, friend, and lifelong mentor lay in a hospital bed dying from cancer. As I sat by her bedside watching her life slip through my hands, my husband came in with roses fresh from our garden. They were beautiful, delicate, peach-colored roses that filled the air with a perfume of hope.

In April, she passed away, leaving me to deal with the hole in my heart and the void in my life. The funeral was beautiful, if funeral's can really ever be beautiful. They covered her casket in a spray of those beautiful peach-colored roses. Then, the friends left. The phone calls stopped. Tears came like a flood every time I went to her house, to tend to the things that needed to be done in her absence.

By May, my grief overwhelmed me. I carried bouquets of those peach-colored roses and placed them by her grave. I answered cards and letters, clipped obituaries and wrote thank-you notes, busying myself so as not to notice her absence.

Not long into June, I decided to create a tribute to this woman who so shaped my life. I dried some of those peach-colored roses and crafted an arrangement to frame her photograph. I worked at the same table where we sat together and said "Grace" over the years. It was a sad place to sit now, in her absence.

When July arrived, the roses were dying from the heat. Maybe they just missed her as much as I did. So many times I wanted to call her and tell her about something funny that happened to me that day, or to cry on her shoulder, or ask her a question that only she would know the answer. My life became a vacuum as I became acutely aware of the permanency of her absence.

August was just as hot, and my soul was still dying like the roses. I felt as if I was violating her privacy, having to go through her belongings. After the estate sale, I stood in the empty house and fully felt the weight of her absence.

A few months later, I had to pick out another beautiful spray of roses for my father's casket. With his passing, my life had become as empty as the rosebushes in the garden that now refused to bear roses. I felt so vulnerable and insignificant on this huge planet, all alone, in their absence.

My life changed as dramatically as the seasons. Even though I was in my mid-forties, I suddenly felt orphaned. And even though my parents were in their golden years, I felt as if I had buried the parents of my youth.

Life is like a precious rose. Every flower is a joy to behold, for it's fragile beauty is only for a short time and then it's gone.

As the seasons continue to change, I realize that life does go on, even though it changes. Still missing them both, I cherish the things they left behind: priceless memories, precious siblings, and a deep sense of their undying love. It's been nearly a year now, and the roses are blooming again as they stand tall and lift their buds to the warm sunshine.

Mimicking the roses, I stand tall and raise my face to the Heavens, knowing I still have life left in me. Thanks to the love of my parents, my roots are strong. Though the leaves may have fallen, I know I still have enough strength left to bloom again.

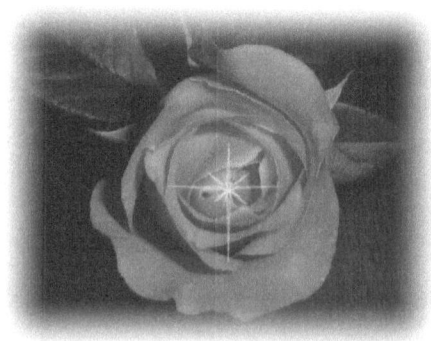

THE BOOK OF LIFE

...and the books were opened,
and another book was opened,
which is the book of life.
Revelations 20:12

Our lives are like Books in God's vast library of time. They begin with our birth and every event is recorded on a line.

As we grow and mature or work through each crisis one by one, we can rest quite assured there's a chapter in our Book that is done.

But if we stumble in the middle and aren't sure of the way we should turn, we can look to the Heavens and know God is trying to teach what we should learn.

For remember that the Lord has already read our Book from start to end. He's memorized each line, so He knows where we'll stumble or we'll sin.

So, if you're stuck in Chapter 12 and feeling torn apart as if it's all in vain, turn your eyes towards the Heavens and lift your prayers to Him, in Jesus' name.

For He's a loving God who say's we'll never have to walk through this Book alone. So stretch your hand to Him and know He hears your every whimper, cry and moan.

Remember when Joseph prayed from the darkness of his lonesome prison cell for God to release him from the injustice of his own personal hell?

Surely Joseph thought this time must have been near the ending of his Book. But if you've forgotten the role he played years later, then take another look.

For Joseph wasn't finished. In fact, his Book had really just began. And God, in His knowledge of the plot, put Joseph in a position to command.

And don't forget the story of all the suffering and pain of poor old Job, who said bravely, "When he hath tried me, I shall come forth as purest Gold."

God takes His gold and melts it in the hottest of any other smelting pot, to make it pure and refined, to be the very best that He has got.

So open your eyes and your heart and reverently take a long, silent look. And keep in mind that God above knows the beginning, the end, and every page of your Book.

HOPE

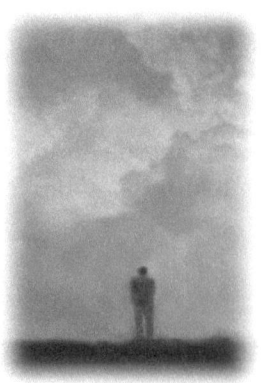

I can hear the storm clouds
gathering in the distance,
growing ever more impatient
with thunderous repose.
Yet, through the small
and secure portal
within my pounding heart -
I hope.

LET'S CELEBRATE!

There is a very special place
where all my loved one's wait.
They reminisce and pass the time
at Heaven's pearly gate.

The streets of gold and mansions there,
(I don't mean to exaggerate)
are beautiful beyond compare
and exquisitely ornate.

I'm telling you the truth, you see.
The fact's I simply state,
to describe for you this holy place
that Lord Jesus did create.

I've missed them, each and every one.
My grief I can't fully state.
So on the day that my time comes
our reunion will be great.

On that glad day up in the sky
I'll join them at the gate
and rejoice when all the angels shout,
"Alas! Let's celebrate!"

WHY?

There are no words to describe the devastation grief causes to the soul. When a loved one is sick and cannot recover, the family is forced to watch them deteriorate. Grief begins it's torment long before the loved one dies.

The days, weeks, months, and in some cases even years of torture, standing by knowing there is nothing you can do to help, watching a loved one get weaker or sicker, watching the progression from a healthy vibrant life to standing in death's doorway, is unbearable. This is the kind of grief millions face every day.

As horrible as this may be, there are other things that multiply the magnitude of grief. A cruel, callous homicide. An unexpected and violent accident. Suicide. The death of an innocent child. These events take a family and spit them into a dark abyss swirling downward to a place that truly only the strong survive.

After the initial shock and disbelief, the loudest question becomes, "Why?"

Why did God allow this to happen? Why did this happen to someone who was so kind, so good, so young? Why now? Why them? The question reverberates in our minds over and over again. We demand answers, but no answers come. The anger builds. The frustration mounts. Even Christians soundly rooted in their faith waiver. Where are the answers? Where is the comfort?

As a Christian, I myself have wondered many times, "Why?" Several years ago one of my family members was killed in a tragic, freak accident. She was only thirteen years old. Vibrant. Giggly. Loving. She had her whole life ahead of her and in an instant it was taken away. Our strong Christian family screamed our own share of "why's" as we searched for some inner meaning.

We tried to rationalized that God was sparing her from some calamity later on down the road. We guessed that God loved her extra special and called her home so she could be with Him sooner. We supposed that He needed her more than we did. We cried that we may never know the reason why, but in our hearts we still longed for answers. It seemed so unfair. So cruel. Sometimes it seems as if the wicked get to live long and prosper, while the good die young. Why?

She had been a good child. She hadn't done anything wrong. She was just in the wrong place at the wrong time. So why did she have to die? Why did she have to die so violently? Why did this tragedy have to happen?

The answer is actually very simple, but so very difficult for us to accept, and offers little in the matter of comfort. But it's the only true answer.

Only God knows.

The creator of an airplane knows the exact workings of each part and what it takes to get that airplane in the air. The average passenger sitting in a seat as it taxis down the runway, doesn't have a clue. But the passenger flies from one end of this country to the next because he has placed his trust in the creator of that airplane.

God is our creator. He knows the exact workings of this life we are living. We are the average passengers, and most of the time we don't have a clue. When things go wrong, we don't know why, only that something terrible went wrong. Our Creator knows why, for He is our Creator - and in His Divine wisdom He knows all. There is nothing He does not know!

There is a reason why a loved one dies and for whatever circumstances occurred surrounding their death. Just as there is a reason for everything else on this planet. God is our Creator. He created the sunshine and the night for a reason. He created the length of the seasons for a reason. He placed the stars and the planets throughout the universe in exact locations for a reason. He is the one who laid the foundations of the universe and he did so for a specific reason. The rotation of the earth, the location of the moon, the distance to the sun - all were created for a reason. His reason.

Job had every calamity known to man happen to him and his family. He lost everything. His family. His wealth. His home. His health. When he questioned God for the reasons why, God responded by asking Job, "Where were you when I laid the foundation of the earth? Tell me, if you know. Who marked off its dimensions? On what were its footings set, or who laid its cornerstone while the morning stars sang together and all the angels shouted for joy?"

In other words, there are so many things we don't know and with our finite minds we cannot begin to understand. For God to explain to me why my cousin died, would be like that aeronautical engineer trying to explain to an infant the complex theories of aeronautics.

We have so many unanswered questions, but God alone has all of the answers. That doesn't help, you say. Your heart still cries for answers. This is where you, as the passenger in this life, need to trust in the Creator.

We get angry. God could have prevented this tragedy, but He didn't. You are right. He could have prevented it. But He didn't. God could have reached His hand down and stopped the truck right before the accident. He could have reached out of the sky and lifted your loved one up to safety right before their tragedy, but He didn't.

Why?

Only God knows.

Everything is according to His plan. Everything. Even though it hurts. So what is His plan? God had one ultimate plan in all of His creation. He created us so that He could love us, and that we would love Him in return, and in that ultimate love, that we should become like Christ. From the moment of our birth until our last day on earth, God continues to be our Creator, sculpting our spirits to be more Christ-like. The day we are born, we are as a lump of clay, and throughout our life He chips away that portion of us that does not resemble Christ and molds us with His hands, so that one day, we will indeed be glorious creations, worthy of the glorious place He has prepared for us.

Nothing happens to us in this life that doesn't relate to His divine sculpting. Nothing. And nothing happens to us in this life that ever takes the Lord by surprise. He knows our lives from beginning to end, even from the moment he conceived each one of us in his thoughts.

When children are born, parents know they have given birth to mortals and they can not live forever. Yet, they still continue to have children. These precious children may live for one day or a hundred years. Parents have no way of knowing that magical number. Only God knows. But it doesn't prevent people from continuing to bring forth children into this world. Even knowing they will one day die, we continue to bring them into the world out of love and hope.

We hope they will live longer than we do, but we know there are no guarantees. So we love them and cherish them as much as we can while they are in our arms and in our care, even if only for a little while. For the joy that children bring to a family is immeasurable. It's truly a gift from God, no matter how long or short that joy may be.

Our task is to love our children as much as God loves us and raise them with faith and values so they will become strong adults with good moral character. Sometimes our task is cut short and God calls them home too soon, long before we are ready. But if we have done our job correctly, there will come a day we will be reunited with these wonderful children. Remember that death is not the end of life, only the end of this mortal body.

Why does God allow a little child to die? Or a loved one to die violently? Or other horrible tragedies? I repeat, Only God Knows. I could guess any number of reasons, but how can I second-guess God? It would be crazier than trying to second-guess the creator of the airplane as to why the whatszit it attached to the whatchamacallit. I wasn't there when he was creating that airplane. I don't have his wisdom of aeronautics. I don't have his knowledge of mechanics. I just want to get to Miami. I don't need to know how it works. I only need to trust that it does.

I wasn't there when God was laying the foundations of the earth and set all of creation into place. Neither do I have His knowledge or His wisdom. I would be foolish to try to guess. I just know I don't have to know all of His inner workings in my life in order to live. I just want to get to Heaven!

Sure, the hurt and the anger are still there. The pain is real. But God's love is also very real, and the one true thing in all of creation is that He does love you. More deeply than you have ever loved anyone, and in ways you cannot even begin to imagine. After all, He is the Creator of love. He knows it's innermost workings.

You may never get the answers you seek in this lifetime. Then again, even if you had all the answers, there is no guarantee that it would offer you one ounce of comfort. Maybe we are actually blessed by NOT knowing all the answers. I often think it's best that I cannot see things from God's perspective. I'm not sure my heart could take it.

The answers will come in due time, though, maybe not in this lifetime. But in the meantime, God will provide you with the strength and the courage to continue day to day as you learn to get past this tragedy in your life. Spend a lot of time close to Him by studying the scriptures to see the answers that are there, and by talking to Him in prayer.

The answers to your questions may be elusive, but the comfort, strength, and peace to get past this - is there with Him.

For I am convinced that neither death, nor life,
neither angels nor demons,
neither the present nor the future,
nor any powers,
neither height nor depth,
nor anything else in all creation,
will be able to separate us from the love of God
that is in Christ Jesus our Lord.
Romans 8:38-39

FROM BIRTH TO BIRTH

Do you remember? It wasn't so long ago when the doctor told you I was growing inside of you. Do you remember the joy and wonder that you felt?

I remember. I was so excited to be making my journey into your world. I chose you, you know. Of all the parents in the world, I chose you. It was quite miraculous really, for both of us. Do you remember the first time I moved inside your womb? My first kick? My first hiccup? You were so happy and full of joy. You sang to me and I heard. You talked to me and I listened. When you moved, I rocked gently inside of you and it was so comfortable. You carried around my picture and showed it to all of your friends, even though I didn't look much like a child, but more like a tadpole. Still, you shared your joy with those around you.

I know you must remember vividly the day I was born. Birth really is a miracle, you know. We enter this world through our earthly parents, coming from the darkness of the womb into the light of our parents love. He told me it would be difficult. He said life on earth is hard and filled with joys and tears. He was right. Of course, He always is. For He created this great world and all that is in it.

You shed tears the day I was born, but did you grieve? Did you mourn? Certainly not! Those were tears of absolute joy! You didn't grieve for an empty womb. You didn't mourn at the loss of the tiny child inside of you. Instead, you rejoiced that the child you carried in your womb, you could now carry in your arms.

Do you remember how many times over the years you held my hand? I will never forget. You held my hand the first day you took me to church and I was afraid for you to leave me in my class alone. You held my hand when you walked me to the bus to go to school. I was afraid then, too. Your hands were so safe when I was insecure and afraid. I will always remember the love and the comfort I felt there - in your hands.

You also held my hand when I was sick, and the doctor told us I would not get well. There was so much love in your hands, but I could see the pain in your face. Life, no matter how long, always seems to be too short. You cry, "Why now?" When would have been a better time for you to say goodbye to me? Next year? In twenty more years? Forty? No, there is never a good time to lose someone you love, and in your heart you know it wouldn't have been any easier to tell me goodbye twenty years from now. If you really think about it, you will realize that time is only in your world, not in His.

You must remember this, for this is the Truth. Do not grieve now for your empty arms, as you did not grieve for your empty womb. I am not dead. I did not die. I was born into your world and you held my hand for awhile. Now I've been born out of the darkness into the light of my Father's world, where He holds my hand.

Remember that grief is natural, but you must not let it control you. There are many joys for you up ahead. He has told me so. The day will come when you will be reborn also, and He will welcome you with His open, loving arms. Until then, He will hold your hand and walk you through each difficult day ahead.

Be comforted in the knowledge that my love didn't die when I left you. It lives throughout all eternity. Lean on Him when you are afraid or when your grief seems to overpower you. Let Him guide your footsteps as you so many times guided mine.

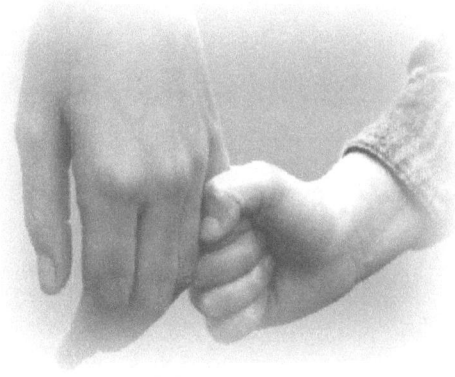

THE GIFT

What can I give you, asked the Lord,
that would bring you the greatest joy?
You asked me for a child to love,
so I'm sending this baby boy.

Enjoy him now and raise him well.
Teach him faith, compassion and love.
Then, let him go when his time comes
to live with his Father above.

You may keep him, but just for a time.
He's on loan from me to you,
as one day you must let him go -
the hardest thing you'll ever do.

Then, one day you will join us here
where joy far outweighs sorrow.
Until then, fill each day with love,
and let Me take care of tomorrow.

COPE
"HOPE" SPELLED WITH A "C"

We all have different ways of coping in life. Some knit, some paint, some play the piano, some just enjoy taking time out to watch the butterflies or the birds. It's a task that we can do without thinking. Something that takes our minds off our immediate problems. A means of escape. Whatever your talents, whatever your hobbies, take some time to relax.

Personally, I write. Poetry and journaling take me out of my turmoil and place me temporarily in another time and place where I can mend. Suddenly, I'm not surrounded by grief, or family crisis, or financial burdens, or stress. I've taken a mini-vacation to another world, even if only for a brief moment or two. But this mini-vacation is worth all the gold and silver in the world, for it helps maintain my personal sanity!

When I can't write and the words just won't come, then I read. It's another form of escape. Reading puts me into a world I might never actually visit personally, or into a totally different time. I can be a part of someone else's life for awhile when mine seems to painful to bear.

Find something you can do without thinking. A secret place where you can escape from your grief, even if only for a few minutes a day. It's a time and place where you can begin to mend. If you don't have a special hobby, or a place you can go for a few minutes, then use a towel. Laugh if you want. Laughter is good for the soul, but the towel works every time.

Many years ago I heard a story of a woman who had six children and couldn't find any time for herself. (I can imagine why!) Every day, she took 10-minutes out of her day and sat at the kitchen table and covered her head with a dish towel. She told her children it was her prayer towel, and when the towel covered her head, she was praying and they weren't to disturb her. It was only for 10 minutes, but it was her mini-vacation escape. She admitted she felt quite foolish at first, but the peace she felt after her 10-minutes of escape was worth all the giggling she heard in the background at the beginning.

I'm not saying you should bury your head in the sand or that any of this will make all of your problems disappear. It's not that magical. But a 10-minute respite each day, even if it's only sitting at the kitchen table with a towel over your head, is 10-minutes of peace you didn't have before. Find some way to escape, just for a few moments each day. It will help to mend your aching heart.

Here are a few other ideas to help you escape. If none of these seems appropriate to your situation, be creative and come up with some of your own. But whatever you choose to do, you must do this for yourself, for your own piece of mind.

Take a short drive outside of the city and view the countryside. Be sure to concentrate on traffic to be safe, but also enjoy the scenery. Or set your alarm clock and arise early enough to enjoy watching the sunrise. Sit outside. Use that quiet time to take in the smells of the early morning and the sounds of the birds singing.

Spend some time playing with your cat. Pets are a wonderful way to learn how to enjoy life again. To them everything is so simple and basic. Don't like cats? How about an aquarium or a parakeet?

Check your local newspaper for upcoming events and visit an art exhibition or attend a quilting exhibit. Go to a garage sale. Check out local galleries and museums for upcoming events. Call your local library and see what special events they have planned.

It's your escape. Do something you've never done before. Or do something you've done a lot, but something that brings you peace of mind while you are doing it. No, your problems won't go away but it will help you to cope. And after all, cope is only "hope" spelled with a "c".

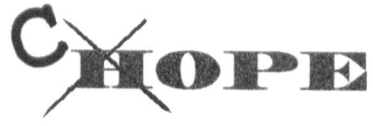

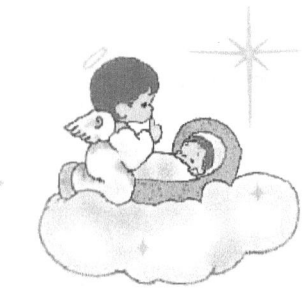

THE LITTLEST ANGEL

I'm only a small child, not much do I know.
God holds onto my hand as I look down below.
I'm here with the Father in the most beautiful place
yet I can't feel much joy when I see your sad face.

Your heart has been broken, I can see from up here
as you struggle along and you wipe every tear.
If I only had words I could send you today
that would tell you I'm home and I'm really okay.

Heaven is beautiful with sparkles and white wings,
and the angels are teaching me so many things.
I'll grow and mature in this Heavenly land
while holding on tightly to my Father's soft hand.

Then one day you'll join me in this home in the skies.
Our joy will be full with no more goodbye's.
So don't grieve for me now but find peace in your soul,
and know God has finally made your little one whole.

Now, even if you can't seem to understand why,
please know in your heart that our love didn't die.
He tells me that just for a time we must wait
and then I can meet you at Heaven's front gate!

I BELIEVE

I believe - that you should end every conversation with kind words and a smile. You never know when you've spoken to someone for the last time.

I believe - that even though you think you can't go on, you really can. It's just that some days are much easier than others.

I believe - that people may not remember what you said or what you did, but they will always remember how you made them feel.

I believe - that heroes are born to every family, and you should always tell your heroes who they are.

I believe - that true friends are the ones who remind you of your dreams when you've long forgotten what they were.

I believe - that it doesn't matter how old you are. You are never too old or too young to be kind to someone else in need, and you're never immune to needing a helping hand yourself once in awhile.

I believe - that the world never stops because your world has been destroyed. The sun continues to rise even though you wish it wouldn't.

I believe - God loves us and grieves when we are sad.

I believe - that nothing is stronger than human ability under crisis.

I believe - that the people you care about most in your life are always taken from you too soon. Of course, anytime is too soon.

I believe - that even when you think you feel so drained that you have nothing left in you to give, when someone cries out to you, you will find the strength to help.

I believe - that God never leaves us. Sometime we just get so overwhelmed by our sorrow, that we forget to raise our eyes to meet His.

I believe - in the power of prayer. That God still listens and cares, and that He still answers prayer.

I believe - that God will never give me any more than I can handle. However, His faith in me is often greater than my faith in Him.

I believe - that life is full of hills and valleys and that both contribute to making me become the person God intends for me to be.

I believe - that five minutes after arriving in Heaven and standing in God's awesome glory, every unanswered question or complaint I ever had in this life will no longer be remembered.

I believe - the answers to every question that is of any importance in this life can be found in the holy scriptures. If I can't find the answer there, then either the question isn't important, or the answer is too complicated for me to ever understand, otherwise God would have placed the answers within easier reach.

I believe - someone, somewhere is looking up to me. As scary as that sounds, everyone is someone's hero. I hope I can live up to being who they think I am.

I believe - if I take things one day at a time and let God take care of eternity, things will be much better off than the other way around.

I believe - hope is more important than love, not just because it's first in the dictionary, but because without it, no other emotion can exist.

I believe - that no matter what happens to me today, there is nothing so great or so terrible that God and I together can't handle it. Truth be known, He can handle it better if I leave it completely alone.

I believe - in miracles. The God that performed miracles in the Old Testament is the same God today, and He is still in the miracle business. The fact that I can still function, even in my grief, is a miracle.

I believe - the best present you can give anyone is a smile. It doesn't cost anything. It can't be refused. It's always appreciated and it softens hearts. A genuine smile can be given to anyone, anywhere, anytime.

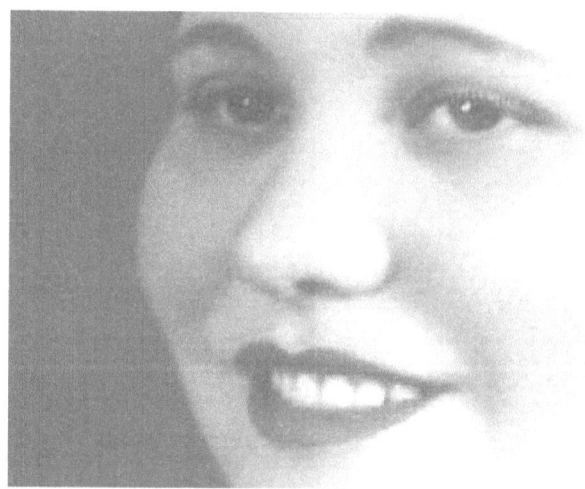

LOST AND FOUND

After an hour of waiting while they worked on her husband in the emergency room, she listened as the doctor said in his grim voice, "I'm sorry, Mrs. Johnson. We used every life-saving technique available, but we've lost him."

While attending church services, she overheard the woman behind her whisper to a friend, "She lost her husband a few months ago. A heart attack. The poor dear."

The friend leans across the pew and tries to comfort her with the words, "I lost my husband four years ago. He had cancer and he suffered for so long. I know what you're going through."

The worship service begins and she wipes a tear as she remembers the day she and her husband were married in the church. They almost weren't. He had been twenty minutes late because he had lost his car keys. Then during the ceremony, he temporarily lost the ring. Looking back now, it seems almost comical. They had lost so many things over the years.

In 1965 they lost their home to a fire, but managed to save their children. In 1971 they lost their family pet, Titus. The six-year-old golden retriever disappeared for four days before returning home. In 1980 her husband lost his job due to corporate downsizing.

She remembers losing much less important things: combs, purses, phone numbers, shoes. Her heart is heavy. Now she has lost her soul mate. Now she is lost without him.

The choir begins to sing louder and the song breaks into her thoughts, "I once was lost, but now I'm found."

A strange peace begins to fill her heart as she realizes the truth. She even smiles. No, he isn't lost. You lose car keys and inanimate objects because they have been misplaced. You don't misplace a loved one. Wiping away her tears, she makes a mental note that the next time someone mentions that they have "lost" someone, she will tell them the truth. They are not truly lost. They have simply gone to live with the Lord, and He has found them.

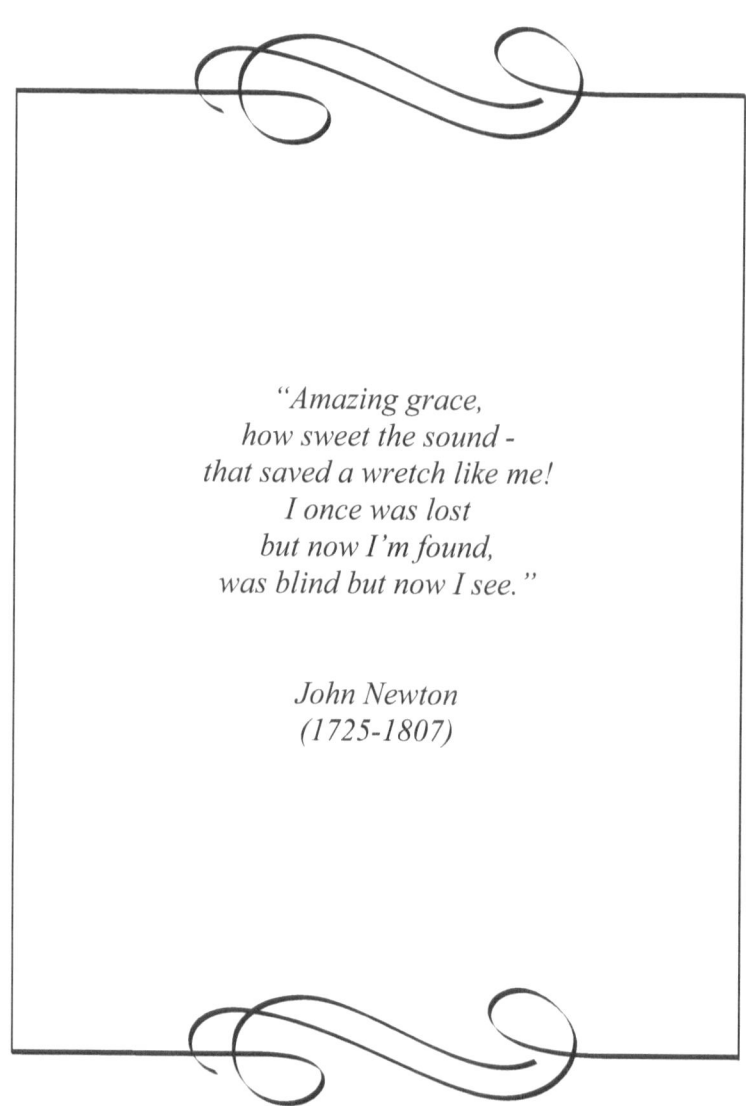

"Amazing grace,
how sweet the sound -
that saved a wretch like me!
I once was lost
but now I'm found,
was blind but now I see."

John Newton
(1725-1807)

WAKE ME UP - I'VE GONE CRAZY!

Dreams are so peculiar. I often wonder what makes us dream. Theologians say dreams can be visions from God trying to lead us through life. Psychologists say dreams are our innermost feelings breaking loose in our subconscious. Scientists say they are caused by nerves and matter clicking together while we are in REM sleep.

I had a dream that got on my nerves, unlocked my subconscious feelings, and gave me visions of things that really matter!

The last two years have been a waking nightmare. While I was in the middle of living a "normal" life, doing routine things like trying to make a living and raise my children, life got in the way. Or at least death did.

Within a period of ten short months, my mother lost her battle with cancer and my father succumbed to a heart attack. Since then, there have been many times my grief nearly overpowered me, and many days my only reason for getting out of bed was to escape the nightmares. Looking back, the worst nightmare is now the funniest.
When you lose someone you love, it's so hard to find any humor. Your grief overpowers every other emotion. Humor is an unknown entity. But I must tell you, this isn't a permanent condition. Humor will eventually return.

I awoke this particular morning feeling like I had been running a marathon. My heart pounded and for a few moments I had to orient myself that I was indeed awake and laying safely in my own bed. Then, as the nightmare remnants began to fade, I began to laugh. A hearty, healthy laugh.

Mother had given me back my humor and blessed me with laughter once again. For in my dream, she was very much alive and very upset with me. You see, she was upset because I had given away her things. No, not the important things, but the useless things she (in real life) referred to as "house clutter".

45

As part of this dream, I had gone through the house, kept the things that were special, in memory of her, sold the furniture and the estate items, and gave away the house clutter. One particular item was a cheap plaster statue that no one wanted. I couldn't find anyone willing to take it. For awhile, I considered throwing it away for it meant nothing to anyone, anymore.

A lady finally came to the door and said it was just exactly what she had been searching for and asked if she could buy it. It was so worthless. It was just something else to dust, so I told her she could have it.

As the dream continued, Mother came home like nothing had ever happened. It was as if she had never been sick, and the main thing on her mind was she wanted to know where all her "things" were. I cried with joy at seeing her and told her we all thought she had died. I was so excited.

She pretended to have no knowledge of the events that led to her death, or the grief I had been going through, and said rather sadly, "Well I really want my things back." I tried to explain to her where everything went, but she wasn't interested. She told me I must find her plaster statue and get it back. Of all the things that were missing, that was the one thing that mattered the most to her.

"The statue?" I cried. "That worthless old plaster statue?"

The rest of the dream is too confusing to try to describe, but the nightmare was a true nightmare. I was lost in my own confusion as I ran from person to person trying to collect Mother's "things" but oddly, no one had kept them and they were lost forever.

Eventually, as the sun rose in my bedroom window, the truth dawned on me.

Nothing on this earth is everlasting. The statue she kept stuffed in a corner of the closet was just as worthless as the priceless mementos in the drawer or the valuables in her safety deposit box when it comes to eternity. None of them last forever and you can't take them with you when you go. You can save what you cherish and cherish what you save, but in the end, they will eventually all turn to dust.

It isn't the "things" that are precious. It's the memories you have of them that makes them so. Memories of the people you love and the times you shared. The "things" are just the souvenirs from those memories.

Still laying on my bed, I thought again of that useless statue. I have no recollection of where it came from, or who had given it to her. I only remember it being moved from one spot to another, seemingly having a lot of trouble finding just the right place. It ended up in her closet because she said it was "just something else to dust". Or something else to turn to dust? She reminded me through this dream that the most important things in life are not "things". That's when the laughter began. Only Mother would use a cheap plaster statue to teach me a life lesson.

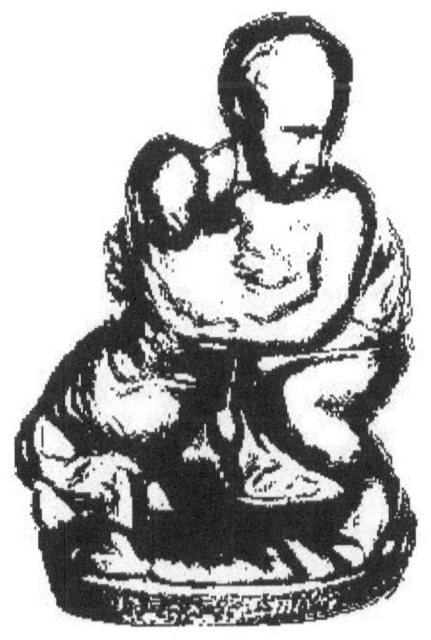

WHERE IS GOD?

She looked up at me with her big brown eyes
and asked me simply, just like this:
"Mommy, I'm wondering. I just gotta know.
Can you tell me everywhere God is?"

She was so perplexed as she continued her query
and she continued on just like so:
"I know I have Jesus down deep in my heart,
but there's something else I gotta know.

I know God's up in heaven watching over everyone,
and I know that He loves us and He sent us his Son,
and gave us a Spirit that fills us with His love
until Jesus can take us up to heaven above,

But, just how can God be everywhere? I mean,
is he here in our house? And is he up in the air?"
I placed my fingers to the lips of this small saint,
and whispered, "There's just no place that God ain't."

THE LAST LEAF ~
A Struggle For Sanity In The Midst of Crisis

The giant leaves turn brilliant hues of red, orange and gold and as the icy breath of Wind caresses them, they curl upward like hands cupped in prayer. Some of them give up early and drop to the earth in mid-yellow while others hold on long after the harsh winter winds have stolen their last morsel of moisture. They hold on through biting winter storms and defy gravity until the springtime buds boldly and somewhat rudely finally push them aside.

Admiring the beauty of the changing seasons, my thoughts ponder the similarity of leaves and people. Some give up early and let life's adversities defeat them. They wither and wilt from just a few tears. Others seem completely undaunted by life's miseries and hang on with unabated strength until the bitter end, refusing to let go until Fate gives them no other alternative. I ask myself repeatedly, "Why do some succeed where others fail? Within what part of our soul, our mind, or our being, does this difference in us lie?"

I learned the difference when I came face to face with my greatest fear: the gut wrenching nightmare of losing a child. Fate put my soul to the mortal test.

From behind the thin veils of Shock and Surprise, I watched the silhouette of Injustice as its icy fingers thrust through my chest and brutally ripped out my heart. The darkness of Despair washed over me. My soul curled from the icy blow and cupped itself as if in prayer as it perched precariously on the flimsy branch of Sanity. My head bowed in Sorrow as uncontrollable tears flooded my face.

"This cannot be!" I cried, as Thoughts raced around me with unanswered questions and completely engulfed me in What, When, Why and How. Unbelief mercifully covered my eyes and wrapped me in a blanket of Chaos and Confusion. I succumbed to the piercing clutches of Hopelessness, and watched solemnly as Strength and Will deserted me. Slowly, I sank down deep into the Mire of Despair. Agony and Defeat pushed me head first into the ice cold Sea of Guilt.

The pain was intense as waves of Sorrow washed me onto the shores of Eternal Sadness. With tears distorting my vision, I realized that I had drifted blindly towards the edge of a great abyss, that great, bottomless Pit of Pity.

I swayed in the winds of Insecurity and felt the thin branch of Sanity slip beneath my feet. Let go or hang on? That was the imminent question. As I scrambled for a foothold, I looked down and noticed a small flicker, like a tiny shard of glass embedded in the branch at my feet. I leaned down and placed my hand over it and it's warmth spread up my arms and into the aching void within my chest.

Realization set in and I knew that this small sparkle was my last flicker of Hope; It had been imbedded by deep-rooted Faith, and as it warmed me I became aware of Strength and Will returning to my side. The branch of Sanity began to grow stronger and more secure beneath my feet. I straightened my shoulders and looked up to the Heavens as the light warmed my soul.

As the tears dried on my cheeks, I felt myself being pulled away from the Pit of Pity. I floated high above the Sea of Guilt until I landed at the moment of Truth. I gathered my wits and glared at Truth with so much anger coursing through my veins, but Truth simply bowed its head and whispered the facts, one by one, knowing that wasn't what I wanted to hear. I wanted to hear that Fate had been wrong, that the torment was over, but Truth only verified the accuracy of Fate's cruel joke and sent the dagger of Despair back through the remnants of my mortal heart.

My only option left was Acceptance. When Strength carried me forward, I laid my shattered soul at Truth's feet. "Then how can I go on?" I pleaded. "Please tell me how?"

Truth leaned into my face and blew its scorching words into my soul. "Because you just can't quit! You simply don't have what it takes to let go. For it's not the things inside of you that keep you holding on. It's the things inside of you that make you let go. Don't you see? Your emotions are all passionate ones, not the pathetic emotions of

Indifference. You're full of Grief, Agony, Despair, and Guilt. Can't you see? You're full of Passion! You don't have what it takes to let the winds of adversity blow you from the Tree of Life: Apathy, Passivity, Indifference or Unconcern. Those are the things that help you to let go."

The winds of Torment blew strong and mighty, but springtime came and found me still gripping tightly to the branch of Sanity. I will continue to hang on tightly until the day Fate gives me no other alternative and tells me I no longer care.

He is like a tree planted by the rivers of water,
that brings forth its fruit in his season;
and whose leaf does not wither.
Psalms 1:3

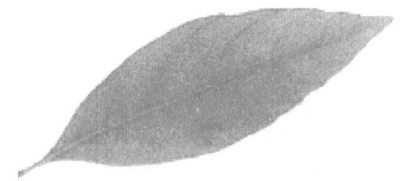

THE HUMAN SPIRIT

In my mind, I cannot imagine living to be a hundred years old. To go from an age of no electricity, to people walking on the moon, microwave ovens, the Internet, and cell phones. It has to boggle the mind living in so many different era's.

My father was born in 1926. He often told me stories of his youth and about times of want. Times were hard in those days. He lived through a lot in his lifetime but worked hard all his life to provide for his family. About the time he retired, technology finally lost him even though he was a very intelligent man.

I remember the first time I videotaped my father. He sat there for a long time watching the camera and waiting for me to snap his picture. He kept saying "Cheese." It was so funny trying to explain to him I wasn't using film, but rather videotape that would even record his voice. It was beyond his comprehension.

I'm not old, but I've been around awhile. I've seen things I never even dreamed of in my youth, and it seems like nothing ever surprises me anymore. Except for one thing. The capacity of the human spirit.

As a victim of a sudden tornado in West Texas, it amazed me how folks who had lost everything they owned would offer help to a neighbor. There are heroes everywhere. Folks who look outside of themselves and their immediate trials and reach out to help those other folks who they deem as being in much more dire straights. Real Heroes.

Recently, this capacity of the human spirit revealed itself again. Working at a local college, one of our students learned his father had died and the funeral would be held in a matter of days. The problem was that the student was from Africa and his plane fare to fly home for the funeral on such short notice would be over $3500. He was devastated and yearned to be with his family during this time of grief.

A local travel agency was able to arrange a special emergency rate of $1600 but he was informed he would have to have the money in less than 48 hours. The boy was still disheartened, for that $1600 might as well have been sixteen million dollars. He didn't have either.

Someone sent a campus-wide email asking for 100 people to donate $16 each to buy him a plane ticket home. The email went out at three o'clock in the afternoon on a Friday when most of us were just thinking about going home ourselves for the weekend. Miraculously, within only two hours, enough money was raised to help this young man get home for his father's funeral - and then some!

This may seem like just another story, but it still amazes me. For I know some of the people in this story. Two of them are undergoing chemotherapy for cancer. One just became a widow recently. One just returned to work from a radical mastectomy. Others are struggling financially. And I'm sure there are many other trials in the lives of these people that no one is aware of. But each one of them looked outside of themselves at the trials of a stranger, and gave from their hearts. It reminds me of my mother's favorite saying, though I don't remember it's origin: "I once felt bad because I had no shoes, until I met a man who had no feet." She was always the first to remind me that no matter what sorrows come your way, there is always someone who has it tougher.

When crisis comes, you will always be able to find that little place inside yourself that is stronger than life. It's what keeps us going when we want to quit. It's what makes us help others when we can't even cry out for ourselves. It's what makes heroes. I'm sure those who gave $16 probably don't consider themselves heroes. That young student probably has a much different opinion about that.

Sometimes it seems as if it's much easier to help others than it is to help ourselves. When grief comes to a friend or neighbor, we automatically jump right in to offer words of consolation and encouragement, lend a hand to help, and offer our immediate support. We ask continually if there's anything we can do to help, knowing there isn't. But we allow our friends time to heal and support them through the process.

When grief strikes our own hearts, we crumble from the blow and stagger under the weight of our own helplessness. We should remember to be as kind to ourselves as we are to our friends. I didn't say we should be as strong, I only said *as kind*.

Be kind to yourself. Treat yourself as you would a friend. Know you have experienced a great loss and nothing you can do is going to change it. Know it is going to take time to heal and allow yourself that time. Show great compassion to your own soul - just as you would a friend. You can do that, because you have that human spirit.

WHATEVER!

Whatever is true, whatever is honest, whatever is just, whatever is pure, whatever is lovely, whatever is admirable - if anything be of any virtue, think on these things...and the God of peace shall be with you.
Philippians 4:8-9

WHO AM I NOW?

I was a thousand-piece puzzle put together
and I knew who I was and why.
The pieces fit together so nicely
as we walked through life, you and I.

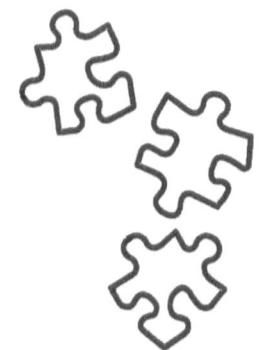

But you've left me and now this puzzle
has been tossed and whirled about.
And I can't seem to put it together
for the pieces are scattered about.

So who am I now that you've left me?
How does this puzzle of me take shape?
The pieces don't quite fit together
not even using glue and some tape.

I wish I had something to go by
like a photo of me all complete,
so I could see if the pieces are placed right
or if I should just give up in defeat.

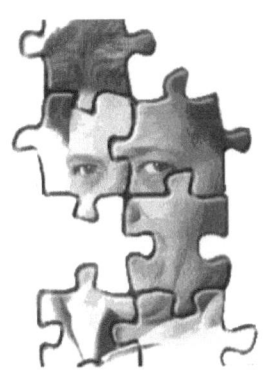

So, who am I now that you're gone?
I know I'm not the same as before.
This puzzle of me is missing pieces.
Critical ones from down in my core.

I'll keep struggling with this puzzle
until I find who I'm supposed to be.
It's just going to take some time
to figure out this picture of me.

Losing a loved one turns your world upside down. Nothing is ever the same again. What was, no longer is. There's an empty plate at the dinner table, an empty chair in the living room, an empty bed down the hallway, and an emptiness in your heart that aches so deeply. It's not used to the vacuum that's left behind when a loved one is absent. Only one thing is absolutely certain: God's love for you NEVER changes. It's my prayer that God will hold you close to His side as you walk through the dark and stormy days ahead, as you search for that "puzzle of you" that's left behind. He will bear your sorrows and give you strength if you only ask Him.

I know this, because He walked with me and carried me through my own grief. God helped me to find my way on this great big planet, using His strength and His guidance. He did this because of His love for me. His love for you is just as strong!

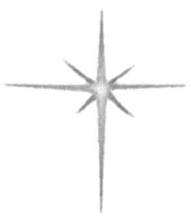

Times change.
Things change.
People change.
God never changes.
God never changes.
God never changes.
God never changes.

Trust in his
unchanging,
eternal love.

MEMO FROM GOD

I see what's going on down there. So effective immediately, please be aware that there are a few changes you need to make in your life in order that I may fulfill my promises to you to grant you peace, joy and happiness in this life. I apologize for any inconvenience, but after all that I am doing, this seems very little to ask of you.

Yes, I know I gave you the 10 Commandments already. Those are good. Keep them. But add these to the list, as they crucial to you right now. I only want to help.

1.
Quit Worrying!

Life has dealt you a blow and all you do is sit and worry. Have you forgotten that I am here to take all your burdens and carry them for you? Or do you just enjoy fretting over every thing that comes your way?

2.
Put It On The List!

Something needs done or taken care of. Put it on the list. No, not YOUR list. Put it on MY to-do-list. Let ME be the one to take care of the problem. I can't help you until you turn it over to me. And although my to-do-list is long, I am after all, God. I can take care of anything you put in my hands. In fact, if the truth were ever really known, I take care of a lot of things for you that you never even realize.

3.
Trust Me!

Once you've given your burdens to me, quit trying to take them back. Trust in me. Have the faith that I will take care of all your needs, your problems and your trials. Problems with the kids? Put them on my list. Problems with finances? Put it on my list. Problems with your emotional roller coaster? For my sake, put it on my list. I want to help you. All you have to do is trust that I am truly in control. Believe me, I am.

4.
Leave It Alone!

Don't wake up one morning and say, "Well, I'm feeling much stronger now, I think I can handle it from here." Why do you think you are feeling much stronger now? It's simple. You gave me your burdens and I'm taking care of them. I also renew your strength and cover you in my peace. Don't you know that if I give you your problems back, you will be right back where you were? Leave them with me and forget about them. Just let me do my job.

5.
Talk To Me!

I want you to forget a lot of things. Forget what was making you crazy. Forget the worry and the fretting because you know I'm taking control. But there's one thing I hope you never forget. Please don't forget to talk to me - often! I love you. I want to hear your voice. I want you to include me in on the things going on in your life. I want to hear you talk about your friends and family. Prayer is simply having a conversation with me. I want to be your dearest friend and believe me, I am listening to every word you say!

6.

Have Faith!

I see a lot of things from up here that you can't see from where you are. Have faith in me that I know what I'm doing. Trust me, you wouldn't want the view from my eyes. I will continue to care for you, watch over you, and meet your needs. You only have to have a little faith. Although I have a much bigger task than you, it seems as if you have so much trouble just doing your simple part.

7.

Share!

You were taught when you were two years old to share. When did you forget? That rule still applies. Share with those who are less fortunate than you. Share your joy with those who need encouragement. Share your laughter with those who haven't heard any in such a long time. Share your tears with those who have forgotten how to cry. Share your faith with those who have none.

8.

Be Patient!

I managed to fix it so in one lifetime you could experience so many things. You grow from a child to an adult, have children, change jobs many times, learn many trades, travel to many places, meet thousands of people, and experience so much. How can you be so impatient then when it takes me a little longer than you expect to handle something on my to-do-list? Trust in my timing, for my timing is perfect. Just because I created the entire universe in only six days, everyone thinks I should always rush, rush, rush.

9.
Be Kind!

Be kind to others, for I love them just as much as I love you. They may not dress like you, or talk like you, or live the same way you do, but I still love you all. Please try to get along, for my sake. I created each of you different in some way. It would be too boring if you were all identical. Please know I love each of your differences.

10.
Love Yourself!

As much as I love you, how can you not love yourself? You were created by me for one reason only - to be loved, and to love in return. I am a God of Love. Love me. Love your neighbors. But also love yourself. It makes my heart ache when I see you so angry with yourself when things go wrong. You are very precious to me. Don't ever forget that!

With all of my heart I love you,
God

BLIND FAITH

As I gaze up at the beautiful sky
an awesome thought comes out of the blue.
The things that I saw up there last night
are still there in the daytime, too.

The constellations in all of their glory
haven't vanished today with the light.
They are still up there in glorious display
and they are twinkling still just as bright.

If I can't see the stars in the daytime
this doesn't mean now that they are gone.
To rely on my sight and only believe what I see,
I can see now that theory is quite wrong.

How can I know that the stars are still there,
if the light of the day works as a blinder?
The same way I know that God's love is real,
using blind faith as my constant reminder.

God's love is as real as the stars in the sky.
Neither light, nor darkness can change it.
And just like the stars that sparkle above,
It's just exactly as He arranged it.

HOLY HUGS

My daughter and my mother were extremely close. The generation gap must have missed them completely, for even though there were more than fifty years between their ages, they shared an unbreakable bond.

After my stepfather passed away, Mom chose to move in with us rather than live alone, and she lived in our home for the last eleven years of her life. Memaw, as she was called by my children, was so much more than just "the grandmother". She was my daughter's friend, and since my daughter was only fourteen when her Memaw died, she had lived with her Memaw nearly her entire life.

There were many challenges to three women living under the same roof, but we adapted, and even though we didn't have what most would call a traditional family, we were a family in our own right.

They became the greatest of friends. In fact, at times I almost felt like an outsider, as there were many things my daughter would confide to her Memaw that she preferred I didn't know. Of course, if Mother thought it was really important, she would find ways for me to find out, but the fact that she would keep those little secrets solidified their bond of friendship.

When Memaw died, the hole left in my daughter's soul was profound. As hard as it was to struggle with my own grief, my heart broke when I realized the devastation it had done to my child.

It's so very hard to help children grieve. For quite some time after her Memaw died, my daughter underwent major depression. She isolated herself and her feelings and when I would ask her questions, her answers came in shrugs and nods instead of words. She spent most of her time in her room alone.

I gave her space to grieve for awhile until I realized she needed more help than I could give her. We found a Christian counselor and she began going for visits. This helped her more than words can ever describe! Not only did the counseling sessions help her to deal with her depression and her inner feelings, but the bond she formed with her counselor seemed to help fill some of the void of losing the bond with her Memaw.

One evening, I was in the kitchen preparing dinner, when out of the blue, she walked up beside me and held out her hand. Caught off guard, I asked her what she wanted. She just smiled and said, "I just need a hug."

It was such a sweet smile, and my heart rejoiced to finally see the light dancing in her eyes once again. We hugged for a long time as I tried to remember the last time she had initiated a hug. Sure, I had hugged her every day, but this was the first time in a long time that she initiated the contact. Then I thought to myself, "I need a hug, too."

Hugs are strange. For when life is the hardest, hugs are needed the most. They are a great source of comfort and support and so much is communicated in a hug that can't be expressed in words. But it's during these times that hugs are the hardest to initiate or request.

Later than evening as I began my prayers, I still needed a hug. My heart hurt. My own grief always seemed to be magnified in the night, and that particular night I needed an extra ounce of comfort.

I remembered the verses in the Bible where Jesus explained to his disciples that although he would be leaving them, God would send His Holy Spirit to comfort them: "*And I will pray the Father, and he shall give you another Comforter, that he may abide with you forever...for he dwelleth with you, and shall be in you. I will not leave your comfortless; I will come to you.*" John 15:16-18

My daughter taught me a lesson that day. I only had to reach out my hand to ask for a hug. As I prayed, God sent His Comforter with a holy hug. His hugs are perfect. His comfort is complete. His peace soothed my soul and reminded me that I am not alone.

MOMMA'S EASTER LILY

Momma had cancer. When she went to the hospital the last time, someone sent her an Easter lily to brighten her room, only moments later to be told it had to be removed to protect her weakened immune system. Convinced in my heart that she was going to come home one more time, I told her I would take good care of it. She would see it again as soon as she was well enough to be released from the hospital. Mother never saw her lily again. My world turned upside down and days turned into months before I knew it. The lily lost its blooms and withered to nothing but dried sticks. After moving the pot a hundred times, I finally planted the bulb outside. "It can either grow or die," I said, figuring it was already dead anyway.

Time went by and I completely forgot all about that lily, until the next spring came and I saw it growing again. It made me angry. Mother couldn't come back, so why did that lily? It wasn't fair.

It bloomed beautifully that season with no help from me. Then the hot summer sun came and it withered and died again. It's been two years now and it's almost Easter again. As I stare out the window at the planter outside, I am surprised to see the lily once again peeking it's green leaves out of the dirt.

Easter is the religious celebration of the resurrection of Jesus Christ. I've known that all my life. But not until today did I realize what resurrection truly means. To die, and to rise again to live. That's what the lily has taught me. As Christ died and rose again, so does this lily. So did my Mother.

I'm so grateful for this flower that honors my Mother on the anniversary of her death every year. For during a time when I would be so saddened, it reminds me that there is a resurrection. That there is life after death. It rises in all its glory, putting on more flowers every year than the year before. Although I still miss her terribly, especially in April, I look at that beautiful flower and have bitter-sweet memories. Memories of a woman who loved me very much and who I loved with ever fiber of my being. I know in my heart she has gone to live with the Lord, and in that knowledge peace fills my heart. For I know one day I will see her again, and I just can't wait to tell her about her lily.

I don't mistreat the plant anymore because I'm no longer angry with it. Instead, I coddle it and coax it and watch the dirt for signs that it's coming again. Just as I believe we should watch for signs that Jesus is coming again.

MEMORIES

Some days I stare at your picture
and my tears just overflow.
I can't explain why I am here
or why you had to go.

But then there are those other days
when I feel your presence here.
Your picture brings me so much peace
just knowing you are near.

Because I miss you every day
your picture sits in this frame
so I can feel you close to me
even though it's not the same.

I'll always hold you in my heart.
Nothing else can fill that space.
Although you're gone,
your love lives on.
I can see if on your face.

HOLIDAY HELL

How do I get through the holidays? Those birthdays, anniversaries, and other special family events that still come around every single year even though you are gone, and only tear at the gaping hole in my soul.

How do I celebrate your birthday? You aren't here and your birthday only reminds me with daggers through my heart how much I miss you. Just thinking of your last birthday makes me cry uncontrollably. How could I have known it was to be your last one? I don't even remember what I bought you for your birthday and that makes me angry. If I had known it would be the last one, I'm sure I would have given you something much better.

My birthday bothers me even more than yours, for you were the one who brought me into this world. We always celebrated that day together and for the first time in my entire life, I'm forced to celebrate it without you. How can I possibly do that? It's like having Thanksgiving without turkey, or Christmas without presents.

Then, what do I do about Thanksgiving? How can I be thankful when your chair at this table is empty? I remember all of the Thanksgiving's in years gone by and now this holiday seems meaningless to me without you. Christmas is even harder. How do I survive a Christmas without buying you a present to tell you how much you mean to me? How can I get through these days without a hug and a smile from you?

I don't even want to discuss Mother's Day. All the world evolves around spending a day in tribute to Mom. The ads on the television and in the newspapers only make me cry. I feel like I no longer have a mother, so how can I celebrate a Mother's Day?

I want to go to bed and pull the covers over my head and pretend these days no longer exist. I want to take a calendar and a big black pen, and cross out the special days that you and I can no longer share. Someone, please wake me up when it's over. I don't want this awful reminder of my loss and the emptiness I still feel in my heart without you. But blacking out the days on the calendar won't make them go away. Curling up in the fetal position with the covers over my head won't bring you back, or heal my heart, or make my loss any easier to bear. It's like taking a pain killer for a toothache. It only postpones the pain. It doesn't cure the hole in the tooth.

Selfishly, I decide to do something that will make me feel better. It won't bring you back, and it won't cure all my hurt. But it does make me feel better. At least, a little.

During special days, I can't pretend you never existed. It hurts too much. So I pretend you are still here. Even if only for a few minutes. It's a little lie I tell my heart, at least long enough to march myself into the store and browse forever through the greeting cards. I find one that says just exactly what I would want to say to you if you were still here. Pretending you are here for just that long gives me the strength and courage to try to find just the right card.

I write a special note to you inside the card, just like I did on all of those other special days. I even sign it, "I love you Mom - Love, Your Daughter".

Then I do something else that selfishly makes me feel better. I cannot buy you a gift to go with the card, for even "Priority Express" doesn't deliver mail where you are. Believe me, if they did I would wrap myself in a box and ship me there for just one last hug from you. But since I cannot buy you a gift, I take out my checkbook and write out a check in the same amount as the gift I would buy for you if you were still here.

My heart is easily deceived, and writing that check helps me to believe that I'm still doing something special for you on these special days of the year. Maybe I'm selfish. Maybe I need this little bit of comfort to help me make it through the day. But these days, I'll take whatever comfort I can find, selfish or not.

I lovingly put your card in the envelope, and then address the envelope and the check to Hospice, who helped us care for you in such a special way during your last days here. Sometimes, I address it to the American Cancer Society, in the hopes that this little bit put together with someone else's little bit can help find a cure so other daughters don't have to go through what your daughter goes through. And so some other Mom doesn't have to go through what you had to go through. Cancer is cruel. This is only a little thing I do to get through those special days, but I know you would approve, and it helps ease the emptiness I feel inside. I also know that these donations help others, even though it's only a small amount I give.

I still miss you and I still hurt, but I try to concentrate on all of the beautiful memories you left behind. It's easier than trying to pretend they never happened. So many women never experienced the joy that comes from having a Mom who is also your very best friend. I consider that to be God's greatest blessing and I thank Him for that every day.

Of all the things you ever gave me, I cherish most the fact that you raised me in a home deeply rooted in faith. It's the most precious gift you ever gave me and I don't think I ever said, "Thank you."

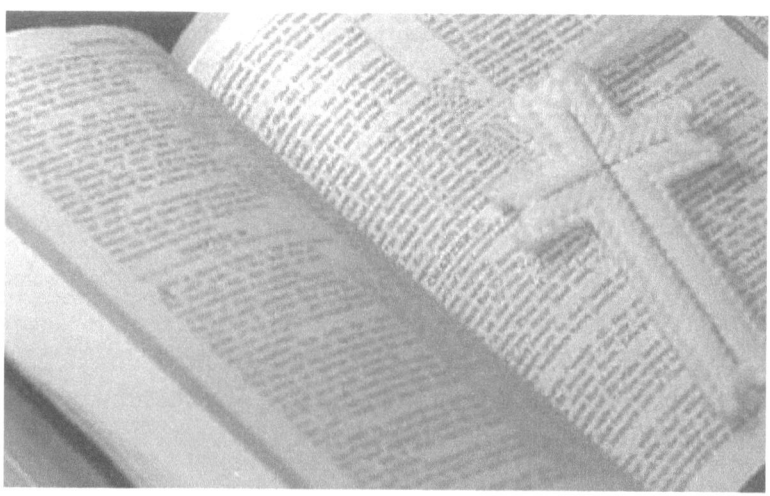

NINE POUNDS OF HEAVEN

I had nine pounds of Heaven
that I rocked to sleep at night,
and I often watched you sleeping
long after turning out the light.
I'm sure the angels missed you
although crazy as it sounds,
Heaven must have felt quite empty
when they loaned me those nine pounds.
My heart is now that empty
and I miss you day and night.
But as I hold onto your memories,
I know now, Heaven is alright.
I'll always hold you in my heart.
'til I once again behold your face
in a Heavenly celebration
when He calls me to that place.

ONE SLEEPLESS MORNING

My eyes grow weary but I cannot sleep
as a million thoughts race through my mind.
I can't smile or laugh. I merely weep
knowing you're gone, and I'm left behind.
I close my eyes and I can see your face,
I can hear your laughter and feel your touch.
But when I open them I see an empty place
that reminds me that I miss you, oh, so much.
The rain outside has finally come to an end
but the rain in my heart continues to pour.
I have many doubts my heart will ever mend.
My grief lies so deeply within my core.
What's that? Did I actually hear your voice?
You see me struggling and it makes you cry?
Did you say that for you I must go on?
It's time for me to live, as it was for you to die?
No, I don't think you fully understand my pain
else you wouldn't dare to ask such a thing.
I don't see how I can truly "live" again
as my aching soul has no song left to sing.
I heard you again, but I can't believe my ears.
Now I know I've gone crazy in my sorrow.
I heard you quite plainly state that my fears
will look better with each new tomorrow.
I placed my hands on the window sill
as the sun's rays spilled through the dark sky.
Without you, my life will be all uphill.
I can't make any promises, but I'll try.
A bluebird flew passed the window pane
and preened quietly on the garden gate.
It was then that I knew I could live again,
and that in Heaven, for me, you would wait.

DADDY'S HANDS

Daddy was a man of small stature, but he had a big heart and big, strong hands. When I was young, his hands were always calloused from hard work, trying to provide a living for his family in the Texas oilfields.

As I grew up, he had big hands to discipline with, and strong hands to hold onto. Any time I ever got into trouble, he was there to give me a helping hand to pull me back up on my feet. Daddy always had warm hands filled with love.

He prodded me with those hands when I was uncertain, he pushed me forward with them when he knew I needed more than prodding. He pulled me back with them when I was foolish, and he held me with them when he knew I needed his strength.

Then a time came when he had a major stroke. His right hand no longer worked as the stroke had paralyzed him on his right side. Suddenly, this man who was so independent was forced to ask someone else for a helping hand. Daddy had been through wars, fought hunger, struggled to earn a living during tough times, and faced many crisis in his life. But the hardest thing he ever had to learn to do was to ask others for a helping hand.

He struggled for months during physical therapy, determined with a will so strong that one day he would regain the use of that hand and be able to stand on his own two feet once again. Eventually, his determination paid off and he did regain some use of that hand, but never enough to suit him.

After he recuperated and went back home, he wrote me little notes that were barely legible, but proved his strong determination in learning to reuse that hand. He was so proud that he was able to write even short little notes that he mailed them to me just to show me how well he was improving. We were both so proud!

As time progressed and he struggled with his own health, Daddy continued to offer his helping hands to others, helping many in ways too numerous to count, in ways that only Daddy could. He had a kind heart. Sometimes, too kind. But he was thankful for his own blessings, and tried in so many ways to help others who were less fortunate. Sometimes he helped in small ways, unobtrusive and behind the scenes. Other times, he just jumped in with both feet and really bailed someone out of a bind.

Time passed by too quickly and the day came that Daddy's heart finally gave out in spite of recuperating from the stroke. I've felt so distraught that death took him so quickly and that I wasn't there to hold onto his hands and to say goodbye. I felt like I had failed him.

He used to joke that he had no friends. He was quite a jokester. He also joked that he was never going to die, but rather he would just live forever, if only to prove he could. Daddy told two lies. He did die, on Valentines Day, taking a piece of my heart with him. But the second lie was visible when so many of his friends filled the funeral home. Each one had a special tale to tell of how Daddy was always there for them, with those great big helping hands.

He never succeeded in learning how to ask for a helping hand. He was too independent. Too proud. But he was the first one to offer a hand when it was needed, and the first one to pitch in a hand and help without having to be asked.

Though I have many memories of Daddy, the one thing I will never forget is the strength and the love in his hands. Now, a power much higher than myself holds onto my sweet Daddy's hands.

...Oh Lord...I am with you always;
you hold me by my right hand,
you guide me with your counsel,
and afterward you will take me into glory.
Psalms 73:20, 23-24

ANSWERED PRAYERS

Did you ever watch a child ask his father for something that child REALLY wanted? They ask with a "Can I? Can I? Can I? Please?" and they are so impatient! Did you ever see their expression when the "Yes" they were anticipating only moments earlier suddenly became a "No"? Teary eyes plead, "WHY?"

It's the same when we go to our Heavenly Father and ask for something we really want. He always answers our prayers, but sometimes it's "Yes", and sometimes it's "No". The answer we're never really prepared for is when he says, "Wait." Many times we cry out, "WHY?"

How do I know God answers prayer? I know because He answers my prayers.

I asked God to cure my mother when she was ill. His answer was "No." But He did answer. I don't begin to understand why he said, "No" any more than a little child who asks his earthly father for something and gets a "No" answer. But I do know that I am the child, and He is the Father. He has all the answers, and He alone knows His purpose.

When I realized she was not going to get well, I changed my prayer to the Father. I asked Him to give her mercy that she would not suffer. He answered, "Yes." I tried to explain this to my brother as we stood by her bedside.

At first he didn't seem to understand. He said, "Where is your God that answers your prayers." I told him I had prayed for mercy. He said, "So where is that mercy?"

That's when I told him to listen. He looked at me like I was crazy. As we listened, we could hear the crying down the hallways of the Hospice Center from others going through the dying process. I asked my brother, "Now, what do you hear in Mother's room?"

73

Nothing. No pain. No anguish. No crying out. Mother rested in peace in her bed, covered in God's wonderful mercy.

After she died, I asked God to give me strength. He did. For without His strength I couldn't have handled my own grief, never the less all the other tasks involved in handling her final affairs. Later, I asked for God's guidance. I had no clue what to do with the rest of my life since He had taken my very best friend. That's when he said, "Wait." For I learned that He knew I was in no mental state to try to decide something as serious as my future in my current state of grief. He waited until I was stronger. Until I was able to look at the world outside of myself with open eyes. Until I was really listening to what He had to say. Then He began to show me the purpose for my still being on this planet.

So remember that He always answers our prayers. Sometimes it's not the answer we want. But it's the BEST answer. For it comes from the Father, who knows what's best for his children. We can't begin to understand the wisdom of the Father, any more than a child understands the wisdom from his earthly parent.

Hang on tightly to your faith and know that He does care for you.

THE BEACH BALL & THE ANSWERING MACHINE

The realities of grief hit at the most unexpected moments. Many years ago when my stepfather died, I watched my mother go through the different stages of grief. I yearned so to help her through it as she seemed so fragile, but I knew it was something she would have to deal with on her own terms. I knew her grief was different than mine.
In time, I believed she was doing quite well until the day I found her sitting in the floor holding a beach ball and crying her heart out. Her grief overwhelmed her but I couldn't grasp the connection with the beach ball.

My mother and stepfather were both photographers and this beach ball was just a prop used to liven up a photo shoot. Why it had suddenly brought my mother to her knees in tears, I couldn't understand. When her tears subsided enough so that she could talk, she explained, "It has Tom's breath inside!" She explained that she had started to put the ball away when she suddenly remembered the day he blew it up, one breath at a time.

I held her awhile, but I never fully understood her pain. Not until after she died and I began my own great struggle with grief. No, I didn't have a beach ball to contend with, and I managed to handle myself fairly well as I went through all of her things and took care of her affairs.

My shock came when I heard my son's voice as he cried out on the answering machine, "Call me back Mom, and please change that message."

I had completely forgotten that she had recorded the announcement message on the answering machine, and when my son phoned and got the recording of her voice, he broke into tears.

It seems like I stared at that stupid machine for hours before I had the courage to hit the "play announcement" button. My first reaction when her soft voice said, "I'm sorry I can't come to the phone right now," was "DUH!"

Then the tears came. I couldn't make myself erase her voice. That's when I fully understood about the beach ball. No, I never could erase her voice, but I did eventually quit playing it over and over again. At least when we had the power outage and the digital message deleted itself.

Grief comes in all shapes and sizes. Hers was in a beach ball. Mine was on the answering machine.

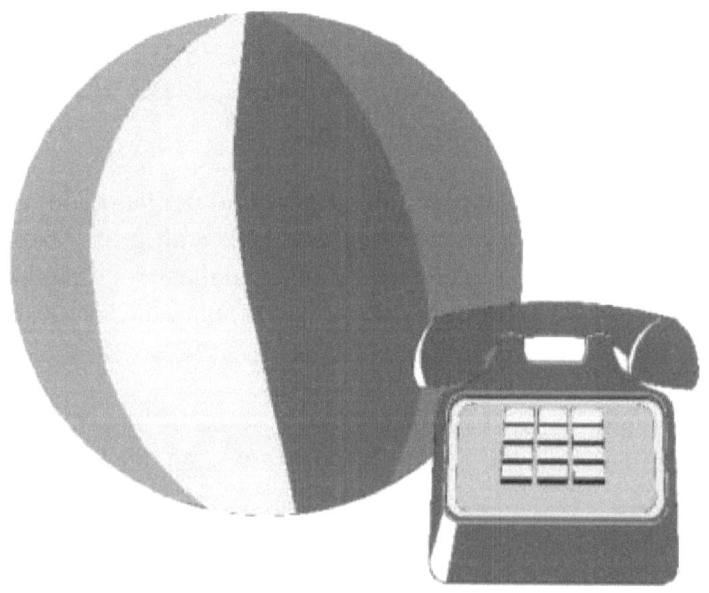

TRADITIONS: NEW AND OLD

There's a joke in our family about how to prepare the tastiest ham. For years my mother insisted the secret is to cut the butt end off before putting it in the oven. I asked her what purpose this serves thinking it must let the juices out to help baste the ham. She said she didn't know, but her mother cooked it that way and it was always the best ham she ever tasted. It became a tradition to cut the end off the ham prior to cooking.

Years later, we were at my Grandmother's house for Thanksgiving and I noticed she "forgot" to cut the end off the ham before putting it into the oven. Shocked, I asked her why she had always done that before, but wasn't doing it now. I just knew she was going to ruin the ham!

She laughed heartily and said, "Because now I have a bigger pan. It wouldn't fit in my old pan unless I cut the end off."

Traditions. Things we do that bring us fond memories of loved ones and happy times. Those warm, fuzzy feelings. Things that warm our heart with just a thought. Until our loved ones leave us. Then, they become too painful to bear. Bitter-sweet memories. Painful ones. Holidays, birthdays, anniversaries, picnics, vacations. What once was joy, now magnifies our loss.

So, should be throw away all of those traditions that used to bring such joy to our hearts? Refusing to participate in the old traditions doesn't stop us from remembering them. In fact, the absence of those traditions usually increases the feeling of loss and abandonment. Yet, to continue in the old traditions increases the reality of our loved one's absence. So what do we do when it seems like we can't win for losing?

Create new traditions! Build on the happy memories of the old ones, but work it into a new tradition for you and your family. If your family always went to the beach on July 4th, then go to the beach, but

77

do it in June. Or celebrate at the lake or in the mountains instead. But start a new tradition.

I still acknowledge the holidays with some of the same family traditions. But for now, I choose not to have ham for Thanksgiving.

THE SOUL SURVIVOR

They say the main reason life is so hard is because it doesn't come with an instruction manual. How can any of us survive without the instructions? It leaves us with no reference when things go wrong.

Life isn't like a computer printer. When the printer malfunctions, you can click on the "help" button on your computer and up pops a magical list of troubleshooting tips. Then through trial and error you test each one until you find the problem, and "poof" the printer starts working again. Or if all else fails, you can call a computer expert to help you correct the problem. In either case, there is help.

It's too bad life isn't like that. Or, is it?

Things do go wrong. Usually when we least expect it. Trouble comes along when we are the least prepared for it. But wait - there IS an instruction manual to help us troubleshoot life. It's called The Holy Bible. Yes, you scrunch your face up and say, "Right! Like THAT'S going to be any help to me while my life is turned upside down." But it's true.

This instruction manual was written by the only true authority on life, the Creator of life, himself. Within it's pages you will find tips and tricks to make it through every life-problem that comes along. Now, it's just like the help manual you have for that printer, though. It won't do you one iota of good if you don't use it. It can sit on the shelf for eons but until you open it and begin to understand life, it's purpose, it's plan of operation, and how to troubleshoot the pitfalls, it's just a dust catcher and maybe looks kind of nice sitting on the shelf.

Within this "help" book are instructions on how to raise children, how to make a marriage work, how to set priorities and goals, and how to find peace and happiness along the way. It's an old book but it's in it's gazillionth printing because it works. If it was full of poppycock, it would have gone out of print years ago. This book even offers "help topics" on dealing with your grief and getting past the despair of losing someone you love. Even Jesus wept.

There is no promise in this book that says if you follow all the directions you will live happily ever after and never face another problem. But there are many promises in this book. God's promises. He doesn't promise a life without trouble. But He does promise that we never have to face that trouble alone!

If you can't find anything in the "manual" to help you through this time of trial, or if you simply can't understand the directions, you can call the life-support hotline. It's toll free and answered twenty-four hours a day, seven days a week: P-R-A-Y-E-R. He's always on call to be there for you. Another promise from God. I bet that outweighs any software support agreement you've ever read. There are directions you can easily follow to be able to get past your grief, and to assure you that you will see your loved ones again in the after-life. For not only is God's love eternal, so are our spirits, and we just need a little preventative maintenance to be sure our spirits are maintained to make it through Heaven's gate. Locate your instruction manual, or if you don't already own one, get one! It's a must-have for living and there is nothing between the pages of that book that will steer you wrong.

When life is the toughest and living is the hardest is when you need that book the mostest. It's a great source of inspiration, a faith builder, and a communication tool to help increase your relationship with your Creator, our loving God.

You may be the sole survivor, but don't be angry with yourself for living. There is a reason you are still here, and you can survive the trials of this life.

Follow the instruction manual for living and become a Soul Survivor. Build a close relationship with our Creator. The only repayment He will ever ask of you is that you strive to love Him as much as He loves you. Life is tough. But thank God that He included an instruction manual. For we are truly LOST without it.

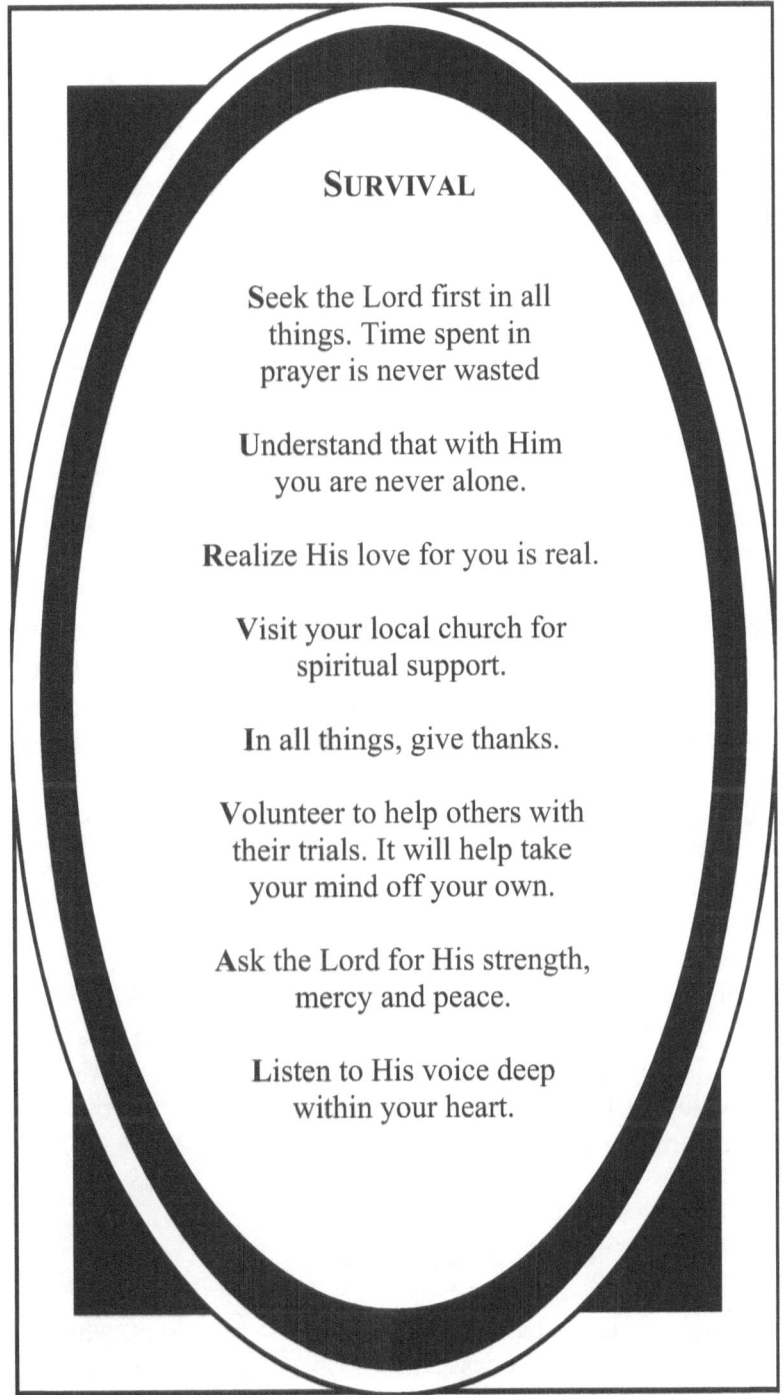

SURVIVAL

Seek the Lord first in all
things. Time spent in
prayer is never wasted

Understand that with Him
you are never alone.

Realize His love for you is real.

Visit your local church for
spiritual support.

In all things, give thanks.

Volunteer to help others with
their trials. It will help take
your mind off your own.

Ask the Lord for His strength,
mercy and peace.

Listen to His voice deep
within your heart.

GARDEN OF MEMORIES

When I was a little girl, my mother was the original recycler. Nothing was ever thrown away. When I outgrew my clothes, any buttons were placed in a box, the zippers put in a bag, and the dress torn into rags and stored in the garage. The buttons would reappear on a new article of clothing later on down the road, as would the zippers. The rags washed the car, cleaned up after the dog, or wiped off a cabinet. Nothing was wasted.

This habit of saving buttons continued for over forty years. Eventually, she accumulated literally thousands of them, all shapes, sizes, and colors. I asked her once what she was going to do with so many buttons. She replied matter-of-factly, "You never know when you're going to need a button." This was her simple philosophy. Be prepared.

On several occasions over the years, I caught her sorting her buttons. She had a drawer filled with neat rows of old flip-top cigarette boxes. In white medical tape across the top of each box, she had labeled them: small white, large red, jumbo black, and so forth. Lose a small green button with two holes, or a light brown one with four holes? One quick glance and she could find an immediate replacement. It usually took her longer to thread a needle than it did to find a matching button.

Cancer began to win the battle over her health. Several weeks prior to her death she became completely unresponsive and unaware of her surroundings. I sat by her bedside day and night on the small chance of her waking up just one last time. It was only then that I discovered the true value of her buttons - to her. One night in the quiet of the room and quite out of the blue, she spoke. Only once. Only one thing.

She said softly, "Oh, I've lost my buttons."

A whirlwind of questions filled my mind. Of all things, why, during this stage of the dying process, did those buttons seem like the only thing of importance to her? Of such importance that it had stirred an audible response from her when nothing else had? It was the last thing she ever said, for only a short time after that she went home to be with the Lord.

Weeks after her funeral, that one statement continued to echo through my mind. Buttons! I went to look for them in her drawer and they were no longer there. Searching through her closet, I finally found them. They were no longer neatly organized and sorted by size and shape, but rather all jumbled in a very large zippered bag in the top of her closet. What a myriad of shapes and color. It was quite an impressive collection.

I sat down on the floor and opened the bag. Never had I ever seen or imagined such a collection. The tears streamed down my face as I pulled out a handful of them and let them sift slowly through my fingers. Mom's buttons. Mom's prized jewels. They were so important to her that she even thought of them in the throes of death. Buttons! I still couldn't understand. What was it that caused this magical hold on her? They were just buttons. Sure, there were thousands of them. Sure, there were some very beautiful ones. But of all the things in life to miss at death's door? Buttons?

As the last few buttons trickled through my fingers, I saw it. It wasn't round like the others and it was very tiny. I picked it up gently with my fingers and just stared at it. Shaped like a bowling pin, about a half-inch long, with two holes in the center for thread, was a black button from my father's old bowling shirt.

In the late 1950's, my father was on a bowling team. I remembered those days vividly. He wore a light gray shirt with short sleeves, black trim, a black collar and pocket and these little black bowling pin buttons. A rush of memories and emotions flooded over me as I remembered the days of my youth. Mother took in ironing in those days to help make ends meet. My senses became so acute that the memories even brought back the smell of her spray starch.

Rummaging through the bag of buttons, I found even more memories. The orange-flowered buttons she sewed on my centennial dress for our hometown centennial celebration. The red apple-shaped buttons she placed on my red and white shirt in the sixth grade. Then years later I used some of those same buttons on a little red summer dress for my own daughter. The purple rose-shaped buttons that had adorned Mom's favorite Sunday dress. The memories were more vivid as I sorted through those buttons than if I had been perusing old photographs.

As I sifted through this color assortment, my heart filled with both joy and sadness. Suddenly, I knew! This wasn't a bag of buttons. It was a treasure of memories! No wonder she kept them for so many years.

I pondered long and hard about what to do with Mom's precious buttons. They were too important to give away or just put in storage. Finally, I knew what I had to do.

The print I found was huge. It's a beautiful print of a large floral garden. A beautiful white gazebo stands in the center, surrounded by trees and flowers of every color of the rainbow. Placing the print on the dining table, I began sorting buttons by color and size. I glued white buttons over the white flowers, red ones, pink and purple, too, over each flower grouping of that same color. The brown buttons covered the walkway to the gazebo and many green ones filled in for the leaves on the trees.

In some of the areas that I couldn't find enough buttons small enough, or of just the right size or color, I filled it in with some textured craft paint. The bowling pin buttons fit perfectly on some of the tree branches; the red apple buttons hang from the trees as if ready to be picked and eaten.

Before this project would be complete, it needed just one more thing. I found a photograph of Mother, trimmed her out of the picture and pasted her in the garden standing next to the gazebo. In her hands, she now holds the floral centennial button. The warmth I feel when I stare at this print now, of Mother in her beautiful button garden, brings a healing peace to my soul. She has gone on, but she left behind a beautiful garden of memories.

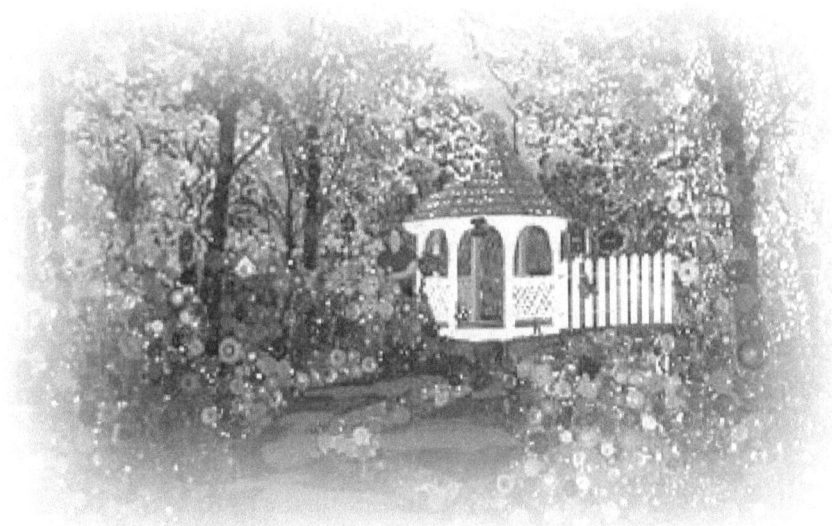

THE MYSTERY OF DEATH

Death is a mystery, only to the living.

I've heard this said many times over the years, but there are two sides to that simple statement. As I continue my journey through this place called Grief, I slowly begin to understand those two different sides.

First, that death truly is a mystery to me, even being soundly rooted in my faith in God. For it involves things unseen and unknown to my mortal mind that I can't even begin to comprehend. Secondly, one day all of the mystery will be made known, as I pass from this lifetime into the eternal one. But not one moment sooner.

Standing in awe of that fact, I recall the many days and nights I watched my mother as she went through the dying process with cancer. It was a long and difficult journey for her. It's odd, the things I can now recall. As her health faded and dying began to take it's place, I spent many hours at her bedside, just watching and listening. It was as if she had one foot planted in this world, and one foot in the other. She wouldn't discuss the things she could see, almost as if it were a special secret. But her facial expressions told the tale of a great mystery taking place in that room.

One morning she opened her eyes and seemed startled, then surprised, as if someone she had known long ago had suddenly paid her a surprise visit. As I watched quietly, she went from initial shock to a broad, beaming smile as she acknowledged her "visitor". She quickly nodded her head as if in answer to a question and smiled again. I saw pure peace radiating from her face, and will never forget the sparkle in her beautiful blue eyes. What joy radiated from her face!

She had many "visitors" over the next few days as I quietly observed. She often reached out to her "visitor". Was she trying to beckon him forward, or needing his touch to prove he was real? Whether you and I believe she was truly visited by someone from beyond, or that she was merely hallucinating, isn't important. SHE believed he was there. I saw it on her face.

Many years ago when my grandfather died, I watched him go through a similar experience, but with one additional detail. His visitor had a name. He called her Margaret. Although he carried on many conversations with Margaret, they were hushed and he muttered so softly that my mortal ears couldn't understand most of his words. He believed she heard him though, as he carried on what appeared to be a two-sided conversation with her. Was it supposed to be a secret from earthly ears? Is that why he spoke so softly? Only occasionally could I hear enough of his conversation to be able to determine that Margaret was his sister. Margaret had preceded my grandfather in death many years earlier.

As we pass from this life, shedding our mortal remains, are we afraid? Does God allow those who have gone on before us the privilege of returning long enough to help comfort us through this passage? Do angels come to us to minister to us during this process? Or do we simply hallucinate as our dreams become a waking reality? It will always be a mystery to us until the day we can see it through the eyes of death.

I watched my mother slowly begin to spend more time on the other side and less time here with me. When I would pry about what she was thinking or what she was seeing, she would simply close her eyes. It wasn't something she felt she could share with me. Maybe it was too personal, or maybe she wasn't allowed to say, or maybe she just knew I would be able to comprehend. Eventually she slipped into peaceful sleep and no longer responded to anything from this world.
I don't know why some people die so quickly, and others take such a long time. Just as I don't know why some people die so peacefully, and others in such wretched circumstances. Another great mystery. Since I can't possibly know all the answers, I will continue to hang on to my faith in the Lord, knowing that on my last day on this earth, all of His truths will be revealed.

Listen, I tell you a mystery:
We will not all sleep, but we will all be changed in a flash,
in the twinkling of an eye, at the last trumpet. For the trumpet will
sound, the dead will be raised imperishable, and we will be changed.
1 Corinthians 15:51-52

REST FOR THE WEARY

Now I lay me down to sleep.
A lesson in futility.
For to put away
the woes of the day,
I don't have that ability.

My wrinkled soul is weary
from this long and troublesome day.
Tied up in a knot
so no matter what,
I'll never sleep, though here I lay.

Why can't I turn off my brain?
Why can't I get loose from today?
Then so suddenly
it all comes to me,
Why, I simply forgot to pray!

Now I lay me down to sleep.
Oh Lord, you know all my sorrow.
Please do your best
so that I may rest
and not worry about tomorrow.

My gnarled soul relaxes
and sleep, I no longer fight,
for He promised me
to hear my plea,
and sends Angels to guard my night.

AN OCEAN OF GRIEF

I cautiously watch the water
as it moves along the shore
creeping closer to the sand
around my feet.

Beyond the crashing waves,
where the water is deepest green
the ocean mirrors the depth
of my grief.

My grief is like the ocean,
sorrow coming in like waves,
sometimes gentle like a ripple
on the sea.

Other times it just engulfs me
with crushing waves of sadness
and undertows of despair wash
over me.

Some days I wade out in it
splashing memories with my feet
recalling days of sunshine
on my face.

Stepping through the foamy edges
never venturing out so far
that larger waves can threaten
their embrace.

Then when I least expect it
this freak of nature soaks me
in reality so painful
that I fall.

The sorrow and the anger
that I've fought with day to day
surge through me in a tidal
free-for-all.

One day when I'm much stronger
and my grief is not so new
I'll swim just like I used to
do before.

I'll take pleasure in the memories,
and tread water in those places
that we can't share together
anymore.

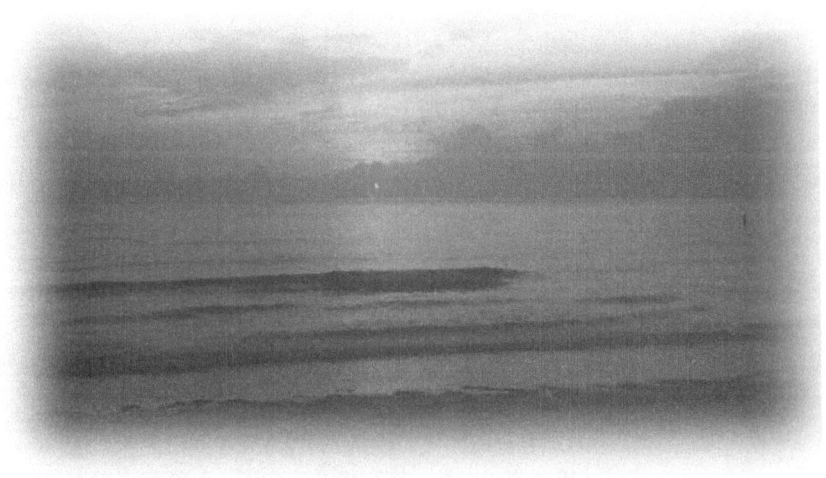

He reached down from on high and took hold of me;
he drew me out of deep waters.
Psalms 18:16

91

THAT HOLE IN YOUR SOUL

The death of a loved one creates a hole in the soul. A hurtful, empty place. An emptiness beyond mere words that seemingly screams to be filled. We try to fill it with positive things but nothing works. We struggle to keep from filling it with despair and anger, but even if we do, it still screams out to be filled. So, what else can we do?

Logic is the basis of the human thought process.

Logic says that if you find a hole in the yard, this means some of the dirt has been removed. So, logically, we get a shovel of dirt and begin to put it back in the hole until it's filled again. The hole is gone. The ground once again is level.

Logic doesn't work with the soul, for logic is a physical thing. This void in our soul isn't physical. It's emotional. Logic is not emotional. So naturally, the logical thing to do doesn't work.

Someone we love has gone and taken a piece of our soul with them. Logic says the only cure is to find someone to love to put in its place. That just doesn't work. Love someone, as it is a good thing. But their love won't fill the void left from a lost loved one. It merely fills a different place - not the empty space.

So what can we do? How can we fill this void? This is where we have to let go of logic and reasoning, and realize that in order to fill the hole in our soul, we have to take something else out. There is nothing you can put in it to fill the hole, but if you take something out, the hole will eventually disappear. Look into your heart and give part of it away. No, that's not logical. But as a result of this, the whole in your soul will heal from within and one day you will realize your emotions are finally level again.

It doesn't make sense. It isn't logical. But it's true.

How can giving away a piece of your broken soul make it whole again? I don't know. All I know is it works. Find some way to give something back to life. Give of your time to an organization that needs your time. Give of your love to a child or an older adult that needs your love. Give of your finances to a person or organization that needs it. Don't give these things in order to be acknowledged for your generosity. Simply give to heal your soul. Give anonymously. Or give in memory of your loved one. But give something back.

Send a "thinking of you" card to someone. Visit a shut-in. Call your elderly neighbor and ask if she would like to go to the grocery store with you. Take some flowers to the nursing home. Call a cousin you haven't seen in thirty years and just say "hello". Send a small donation to Hospice, or a charity of your choice. They appreciate any amount you can send. Send $10 in cash anonymously to a friend you know that needs a special treat. Give away a part of yourself privately simply by putting others on your prayer list and praying for them daily.

I don't know "how" this works. I only know it works. I found out quite by surprise myself. The void was so devastating, I couldn't imagine how I could heal by giving more of my soul away. I couldn't even believe there was anything left inside of me to give, for I felt so empty. Then one day, I was reading a list of messages posted at an online grief recovery website. Touched deeply by the heart wrenching notes posted there, I realized how much grief is truly in this world. Not just MY grief.

I started off by sending an email to a couple of the people who had posted messages there, simply saying, "My heart goes out to you. I too am grieving, but I will keep you in my prayers." The response was overwhelming. No, not their response. MINE! Yes, I received heartfelt notes from many of them and they were so grateful for an ounce of support, but the biggest response was in the healing of my own soul - simply by giving a tiny portion of it away. Over time, I created Rainbow Faith, a Christian grief ministry with a website for those online, hurting, and seeking some form of comfort and encouragement. No, I never pictured myself doing something like this. It just happened. But the healing it has brought to my own soul is miraculous and beyond words.

GOOD VS. EVIL

Evil exists. It showed itself in America on September 11, 2001. Evil has but one mission: to destroy Good.

It's an old story, this war between Good and Evil. The scriptures tell of some of the battles. The news tells of others, both here and abroad. On September 11th we saw its face first hand and it's very real. It's Evil. It's merciless.

It kills Good people. It destroys Good families. It mains Good nations. This unmerciful thing called Evil.

Is there hope? Can Good truly win against Evil? The answers can be found in the scriptures:

> *"All things work for Good for those that love the Lord."*

But what does this scripture really mean? It means that ALL things can only result in GOOD things for those that love the Lord. Yes, even EVIL things. For if we love the Lord, even Evil will result in Good.

Our loss, our pain, and our despair blind us. We cannot see beyond our pain for it's too fresh, too close, too painful, too deep, too devastating. But God can. He knows the final outcome. He knows the end of this war. He knows Good will win in the end. He PROMISES us Good will win. He sent his own Son to die as a seal to that promise to us.

The days are dark. The pain is deep. The hurt is overwhelming. I don't know the "why" of all of this, but I trust in God's promises and believe that Good will come in the end. Hang on tightly to your faith. Be fervent in your prayers. Seek God's face and his peace that surpasses all human understanding. Study the scriptures and read about God's many promises.

DON'T FORGET TO LAUGH

Grief hurts. The emotional roller coaster ride of grief takes it toll and leaves me feeling bruised and empty inside. Humor is a fleeting thing, something I can vaguely remember, but no longer feel. However, I am reminded of the saying that laughter is good for the soul, so I begin to ask myself, "How can I laugh? Where is my joy?" I can find nothing funny anymore.

When my mother died, I lost my sense of humor. It seemed inappropriate that anyone could be having fun when I was going through the most difficult days of my life. Then I realized that humor is required to survive. Survival is one of the biggest reasons God created humor.

Most things make me cry. Or make me angry. But humor is good for the soul and I believe everyone should try to find some humor somewhere to help in the healing process. When we are grieving, laughter comes in the strangest places, at the strangest times. And I'm sorry to say, my first chuckle was while preparing to attend my mother's funeral, and my biggest laugh was at my father's funeral less than a year later. As perverse as that may sound, it reminded me that even though I was going through dark days, I still had the capacity to laugh.

My parents had been divorced for over 25 years but had remained friends for the sake of us kids even though we were grown. When Mother died, my father drove from Florida to Texas to be by his children's side as we buried our mother.

Now, Dad was very parsimonious throughout his lifetime, at times nearly to a fault. Mom and I used to joke about how he would cut corners and pinch pennies, but this was something he had lots of practice at, and did very well.

When it was time to get dressed for Mom's funeral, Dad came walking out of the bedroom in a very nice black tuxedo. Not a suit. A tuxedo. Complete with a silk red rose pinned to the breast pocket. I was surprised to say the least.

When I asked him about the tuxedo, he grinned a smile a mile wide and strutted to show it off. He beamed, he was so proud! Then he told me he bought the tuxedo at Goodwill Industries for ten dollars. Well, he finally admitted it only cost him seven dollars, but he had to pay three dollars to have it dry cleaned.

He was so proud of his savings, that I couldn't say anything to hurt his feelings, so he wore his "suit" to the funeral. Now, Dad made good money all his life, and it's not like he couldn't afford a nice suit, but this is what he wore - and so very proudly at that! He looked so funny, this little man wandering amidst the crowd of mourners, dressed in his little penguin suit, his ten dollar tuxedo. I couldn't help but chuckle - even in my grief.

It was a difficult time over the next several months trying to find humor, but I kept searching, for I discovered that laughter did, indeed, help to heal my aching heart. It was a fleeting thing, and so hard to find, but I tried hard to keep a sense of humor about things. They say it takes more muscles to cry than it does to laugh, but I say laughing doesn't give you a runny nose like crying, and crying doesn't help my heart as much as laughter does.

When my father died, I flew to Florida to assist my brother with the funeral arrangements. We struggled over what clothes to bury Dad in. Do we go out and buy a suit when he wouldn't buy one in life? Do we bury him in his khaki's that he wore everywhere, which were mostly now old and worn?

We worried over it for awhile and finally decided to do what we thought Dad would want us to do. We decided to bury him in his ten dollar tuxedo. We did splurge, however, and went to the discount store and bought him a brand new white shirt to go with the tux. I know Dad probably would have cringed at that, but we thought it was the least we could do.

During the visitation at the funeral home, we struggled with mixed emotions ranging from sorrow, to holding back a chuckle over that silly tuxedo. I was surprised when one of his dearest friends plucked a rose from a wreath and replaced the red silk flower in Dad's breast pocket. She said with a smile, "If he's going to heaven in a tux, he needs a real flower."

Then the laughter came. She and I laughed so hard we cried, or maybe we laughed and cried, or maybe the laughing was to hide the crying, but either way, it was good for the soul and helped to cleanse both our hearts.

Later, I wanted so badly to call Mom and tell her we just laid Dad to rest in his ten dollar tuxedo. It made me miss her even more for she was no longer just a phone call away. Although I still grieved so much for her, and was having to deal with the loss of my father so soon afterwards, the humor of the occasion sure helped get me through the crisis of two funerals in one year.

Betty Eaton, a dear friend, commented that "laughing and crying are close sisters, living together although at odds. Both are healing and uplifting and are similar in both sound and facial expression. Tears of laughter, with the mouth turned upward, are expressing great joy and mirth. Tears of sadness, with the mouth turned downward, are expressions of grief, sorrow, loss, etc., but both are God-given responses and are to be used as He wants us to."

I thank God daily for humor and for the emotional release laughter allows, as well as for good friends and family to share it with. I also thank Him for friends who allow me to laugh. It's not required that I spend every moment of the rest of my life in sorrow. It's also not in God's plan that I do that. It doesn't mean I'm not still mourning my loss. It doesn't mean I don't still feel deep sorrow. For those emotions are still just beneath the surface. It only means I'm using the gifts God gave me, and one of those gifts is laughter.

Grief hurts. Laughter doesn't.

HE GAVE IT ALL AWAY

God gave each of us a talent.

Poppa's gift was helping others.
    Whether it was helping children grow,
    or helping someone laugh,
    or helping those he cared for so deeply just try to survive life,
    he was a helper.

In order to help others, he gave a piece of himself away.
    Whether it was his time,
    his pranks and practical jokes,
    his wisdom,
    or his belongings.
    He gave everyone he knew a piece of himself.

Poppa had a big heart.
    He loved.
    He laughed.
    He joked.
    He gave.

Over the years he gave everyone he met a different piece of his great big heart. I find it fitting that on Valentine's Day, Poppa gave what was left of his heart
    to God,
    to go home to be with his thirteen brothers and sisters,
    his parents and grandparents,
    and many friends who have gone on before him.
    I'm sure he's sharing with them all the love he experienced on this earth. He's surely telling about his family,
    and his life here on earth,
    both the sorrows and the laughter.

I now know for certain there is laughter in Heaven.

FIRST AND LAST

When my daughter was born, I bought a baby book that has space in it for recording all of baby's "first's". Over the years, I recorded first words, first steps, first tooth in and first tooth out, and many other first's. Since I know the mind is the first thing to go, these are precious moments I never want to forget.

It's funny how even now I can read the pages of that baby book and have difficulty remembering the actual events, but I remember how important they seemed at the time!

I vividly remember her first report card, first birthday, first date, and her first job. And now as she embarks on her first (and only, I hope) marriage, I find myself reminiscing about all of the first's in my life. As the first's race around in my head, I'm suddenly reminded of the last's.

The last's are a peculiar thing, for you never know they are the last when they are happening. You only come to realize they were the last, long after they are over.

I remember the last time I carried her to bed after she had fallen asleep on the sofa watching television. I didn't know it was the last time, or I'm sure I would have walked much slower, cherishing the moments as I lingered over her and tucked her underneath her warm covers. At some point, she became too heavy for me to carry, and those walks down the hall with her limp in my arms and snuggled to my breast were gone.

The last time I saw my father, he had driven 1,100 miles from his home in Florida to my home in Texas to be with me for my mother's funeral. As he prepared to leave, I walked with him to the car, hugged him and watched him get in and drive away, waving until he was out of sight.

Did I know it was going to be the last time? No. For if I had known, I would have hugged longer, cried harder, and begged him to stay even if just for a few more days. But I didn't know. Sure, I had plans to go visit him soon. Sure, I talked to him on the telephone every Sunday. But no, I had no way of knowing that in less than ten months, he too would be gone. Neither of us could have known that.

I didn't have a book to record his last visit or our last hug, but my heart remembers it vividly. Other last's, I don't remember as vivid, but wish I could. I wish I could remember Mother's last birthday, and many other last's that passed long before I realized. Once my parents were gone, their last's began to haunt me.

God knows all the first's and the last's. I suppose it takes a Divine heart to be able to know the last of something and not spend a lifetime fretting over it. It's a good thing we don't know when the last of something is occurring, for it would surely break our heart.

It would be nice if we could live one moment at a time, and live each one as if it were a last moment, relishing each hug as if it might be the last, each conversation as if it might be also. Life makes us busy. We each have the same number of hours in each day, but we seem to cram too much in it. More time for working, less time for hugging.

When a loved one dies, it somehow puts everything else into perspective. The things that used to seem so important and time-demanding, now seem like useless clutter. The words said, the deeds done, the kindness showed, and the love shared becomes all important.

As I continue along grief's long journey, even several years after their death, I remind myself of the important things in my life. I linger longer in conversations, hug my loved ones and friends more, and cherish the little things that may soon be last's.

My daughter and I are spending lots of time planning her wedding. She is so excited! I'm excited for her, but also saddened for I know there is another last coming. I hope I know it when it happens. But as I dread the last's, I also look forward to even more first's. For it is in our first's that God gives us our greatest joys and provides us with our greatest blessings.

As you work your way through your own grief, recalling the many last's, remember that God still has many joys left for you, and many more first's. Part of the grief process is in remembering the last's, but treat them like photographs. Cherish them, dwell on them for awhile, then place them away in a special place.

My grief has been like that baby book. I have gone back through the book, rejoiced at the first's, cried over the last's, and now it's time I close that book and get on with life.

It's time to start a new book, for the little baby is gone, but the bride is beautiful!

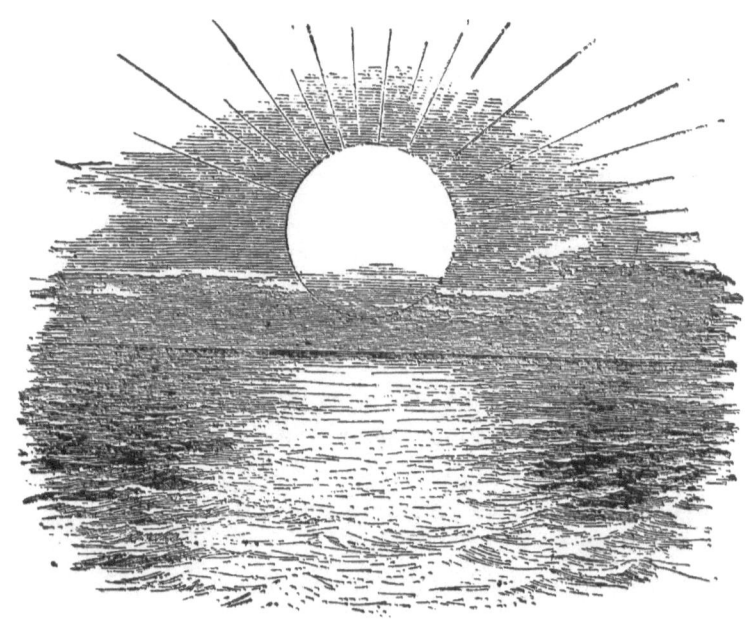

I am the Alpha and the Omega,
the First and the Last,
the Beginning and the End.
Revelation 22:13

Prayers & Promises

As I have stated repeatedly in this publication, the most important thing you can do to heal your aching heart, is to hang on tightly to your faith and PRAY. To help you through the days ahead the following Prayers & Promises can serve as prayer starters for you. They are not designed to be your only prayer, but to only help in getting you started.

My father was the world's worst when it came to following prescriptions. He believed if a teaspoon would make you well, then a tablespoon would make you well quicker! Unfortunately, he often suffered the consequences of overdoing his prescription. However, this prescription for prayer to help you through the healing process of grief uses the very same philosophy of my fathers. And this prescription works best when you DO overdo. A little prayer works. But a lot of prayer works wonders. So use these as prayer starters, and spend plenty of time in prayer. Your aching heart needs it.

Take things one day at a time. Start with the first prayer. At the end of the month, simply start this list over again. You will have made it through the first month taking things one day at a time. Now you can take things one month at a time. After only twelve of those, you can begin to look at healing one year at a time. Time gives you the space in which to heal. Prayer will get you through this time.

Sometimes, it's too hard to pray. The words in your heart tend to turn into tears in your eyes and they never make it past your lips. These are the times when you simply need only to pray with your heart. Be still and listen for God, seeking him with all your heart. He knows your sorrow before you even utter one word. Let him hear your heart and comfort you in ways that only He can do.

May God bless you and strengthen you on your journey, giving you His peace, strength, and divine comfort as he lights your path and plants special blessings along your way.

PROMISE

God is not a man that he should lie.
Does he speak and then not act?
Does he promise and not fulfill?
Numbers 23:19

PRAYER

Lord, help me to remember that your promises are true and eternal. Times change, things change and people change, but you NEVER change. Thank you for your unchanging, eternal love for me.

PROMISE

The Lord is not slow in keeping his promise,
as some understand slowness.
He is patient with you.
2 Peter 3:9

PRAYER

Lord, help me to understand that your timing is not the same as mine. I cannot see things from your viewpoint or your timetable, for I do not have the wisdom to comprehend the mind of God. Help me to trust in your promises.

PROMISE

God is our refuge and our strength,
an ever present help in times of trouble.
Psalms 48: 1-3

PRAYER

Lord, I lean on your promise to be ever present, especially now during this time of sorrow in my life. Give me the strength to move on as you wrap your loving arms around me. Let me take refuge in your love.

Ferna Lary Mills

PROMISE
Though he stumbles, he will not fall,
for the Lord upholds him with his hand.
Psalms 37:24

PRAYER

Lord, my burdens are great. Help me to lean on you, for your strength will see me through these days. Reach down and hold me up with your hand according to your promise.

PROMISE
Come to me, all you who are weary and burdened,
and I will give you rest.
Matthew 11:28

PRAYER

Lord, I am weary and have found no rest. I come to you for your promise of rest. Grant me peace that I may sleep as you send your angels to restore my soul. Nurture my aching heart, Lord, and may I awake refreshed with your spirit.

PROMISE
Let us hold unswervingly to the hope we profess,
for he who promised is faithful.
Hebrews 10:23

PRAYER

Lord, my world has turned upside down. What was before, no longer is, and I'm lost and hurting. Strengthen me as I continue to hope in you. Thank you for being steadfast in your promises.

PROMISE

For God so loved the world
that he gave his one and only Son,
that whoever believes in him
shall not perish but have eternal life.
John 3:16

PRAYER

Lord, thank you for giving me the greatest gift of all - the gift of eternal life. Help me to remain steadfast in my faith and to lean on your promise that life is eternal and death of the body is not a death of the spirit.

PROMISE

I have come into the world as a light,
so that no one who believes in me
should stay in darkness.
John 12:46

PRAYER

Lord, shine your light so that I may find my way. Let me seek you in all things. Help me to trust in your promise: because I believe in you I will not have to stay in this darkness.

PROMISE

For he has not despised or disdained
the suffering of the afflicted;
he has not hidden his face from him
but has listened to his cry for help.
Psalms 22:24

PRAYER

Lord, according to your promise, hear my cries. Comfort my aching heart and lift my spirit up to you to be nurtured and healed in ways known only to you.

105

Ferna Lary Mills

PROMISE
He will wipe every tear from their eyes.
Revelation 21:4

PRAYER
Lord, I cry out to you in my distress. As you promised, wipe the tears from my eyes and give my aching heart the fullness of your joy. Thank you for walking with me through these difficult times and help me to walk closer to you in both the good times and the bad.

PROMISE
For men are not cast off by the Lord forever.
Through grief, he will show compassion,
so great is his unfailing love.
For he does not willingly bring affliction or grief
to the children of men.
Lamentations 3:31-33

PRAYER
Lord, thank you for your unfailing love and for your compassion for me, especially during this time of my greatest sorrow. Let me lean on your promises to make it through the days ahead as you restore peace to my soul.

PROMISE
I have told you these things, so that in me you may have peace.
In this world you will have trouble.
But take heart! I have overcome the world.
John 16:33

PRAYER
Lord, help me to trust in your promise of peace as I journey through this world and the trials of this life. For I know there is no peace but in you, and your peace is perfect.

PROMISE

Then you will call, and the Lord will answer;
you will cry for help, and he will say:
Here I am.
Isaiah 58:9

PRAYER

Lord, you promise to hear my cries and to answer and comfort me. Teach me to be still and to hear your voice even in the gentle stillness and on gentle breezes. I seek you, Lord, to comfort my heart.

PROMISE

He gives strength to the weary and increases
the power of the weak.
Isaiah 40:29

PRAYER

Thank you, Lord, for the promise of your strength and power when I have none left of my own. Teach me to lean on you when I am weak, that I may learn to lean on you when I am strong.

PROMISE

Though I walk through the valley
of the shadow of death,
I will fear no evil,
for you are with me;
your rod and your staff, they comfort me.
Psalms 23:4

PRAYER

Lord, you never promised life without sorrow, but you promised I would never have to go through it alone. Thank you, Lord, for walking through this valley with me and for comforting me along the journey.

PROMISE

No eye has seen, no ear has heard,
no mind has conceived
what God has prepared for those who love him.
1 Corinthians 2:9

PRAYER

Lord, thank you for your faithful, eternal love for me. Help me to see beyond today and to know that the things you have promised me are so far greater than my mind can ever comprehend.

PROMISE

Do not be fearful;
do not be discouraged,
for the Lord your God will be with you
wherever you go.
Joshua 1:9

PRAYER

Lord, let me feel your presence. Let me be comforted even in the silence and the stillness, just knowing you are with me always, even as you promised. Thank you for always being with me wherever I am and whatever I'm going through.

PROMISE

Your word is a lamp to my feet
and a light for my path.
Psalms 119:105

PRAYER

Lord, help me to understand that this lamp may light only a few steps at a time, and that I don't need to see the entire journey. I only need to have the faith to take one step at a time. Thank you for the light, Lord, to help me through this darkness, as you show me your direction for my life.

PROMISE

I tell you the truth, if a man keeps my word,
he will never see death.
John 8:51

PRAYER

Lord, thank you for your promise of eternal life. Though death may consume the body, I know my spirit and those of my loved ones lives on with you forever and ever. In this promise, I can rest assured I will be reunited with them again!

PROMISE

Because he loves me, says the Lord,
I will rescue him;
I will protect him,
for he acknowledges my name.
Psalms 91:14

PRAYER

Lord, some days I need protection from myself. According to your promises, please protect me from my own anger, guilt, sadness, and sorrow. Help me to lean on you and to trust in your promises.

PROMISE

The Lord is an everlasting God.
He will not grow tired or weary.
Isaiah 41: 28-29

PRAYER

Lord, I am blessed by knowing that no matter how tired or weary I may become, you will always be strong. Your strength is sufficient for me as you carry me through the days when I am so weak. Refresh my spirit and help me to continue to trust in your promises.

PROMISE
Call to me and I will answer you
and tell you great and unsearchable things
you do not know.
Jeremiah 33:3

PRAYER
Lord, you promise to hear my prayers and to grant me understanding. I call out your name and listen for your still voice. Help me to understand your will for my life and to trust you with all my heart and soul.

PROMISE
Cast all your cares on the Lord, for he cares for you.
And the God of all grace will himself restore you
and make you strong, firm and steadfast."
1 Peter 5: 7, 10

PRAYER
Lord, you have heard my prayers. According to your promise, I thank you for making me strong, firm and steadfast, even in my trials. I know that all of my strength comes from you.

PROMISE
For he will command his angels concerning you
to guard you in all your ways.
Psalms 91:11

PRAYER
Lord, according to your promise, please send angels to protect me from danger. Most of my danger lies within my own heart: sorrow, pity, anger, fear and distress. Renew my spirit and make me whole again so that I may have true peace.

PROMISE
Never will I leave you.
Never will I forsake you.
Hebrews 13:5

PRAYER

Thank you, Lord for your promise to remain with me through all of my good times as well as my bad. Help me to trust in your promise that you are always with me, every day, every moment, everywhere.

PROMISE
For what I have said,
that will I bring about.
Isaiah 46:11

PRAYER

Help me Lord to understand that the promises you made thousands of years ago, still hold true today - for ME! Thank you for your promise of faithfulness.

PROMISE
Whether you turn to the right or to the left,
your ears will hear a voice behind you, saying,
"This is the way; walk in it."
Isaiah 30:21

PRAYER

Lord, when I'm lost and can't find my way, you promise to lead me. Help me to become a better listener, Lord, so that I may walk in your ways. Help me to shut out the noise of this world and it's woes that I may be better able to hear your still, small voice within my aching heart.

PROMISE

Now we know that if the earthly tent we live in is destroyed,
we have a building from God,
an eternal house in heaven,
not built by human hands.
2 Corinthians 5:1

PRAYER

Lord, thank you for your promise of eternal life. Although death may take the body, I know in my heart that the spirit lives on with you in a place where there is no sorrow.

PROMISE

I can do all things through Christ
who strengthens me.
Philippians 4:13

PRAYER

By your strength alone, Lord, do I continue to function, for my strength is gone. Thank you for your promise to strengthen me in my weakness. Thank you for being my strength and my refuge.

PROMISE

I will instruct you and teach you
in the way you should go.
I will guide you with my eye.
Psalms 32:8

PRAYER

Lord, as you promised, lead me and guide me, for my own sense of direction is blinded. My own eyes are dull and full of tears. Let me be reminded that for you to guide me, you must first be with me, and I know you are with me every moment of every day.

PROMISE

But I will see you again and you will rejoice, and no one will take away your joy. ~ John 16:22

PRAYER

Lord, help me to remember that my sorrows are only temporary in your grand scheme of things. Help me not to be angry and to trust in your promises of the joy that awaits me. It's so hard for me to imagine a time that joy will once again return to my heart, but I lean on your promises.

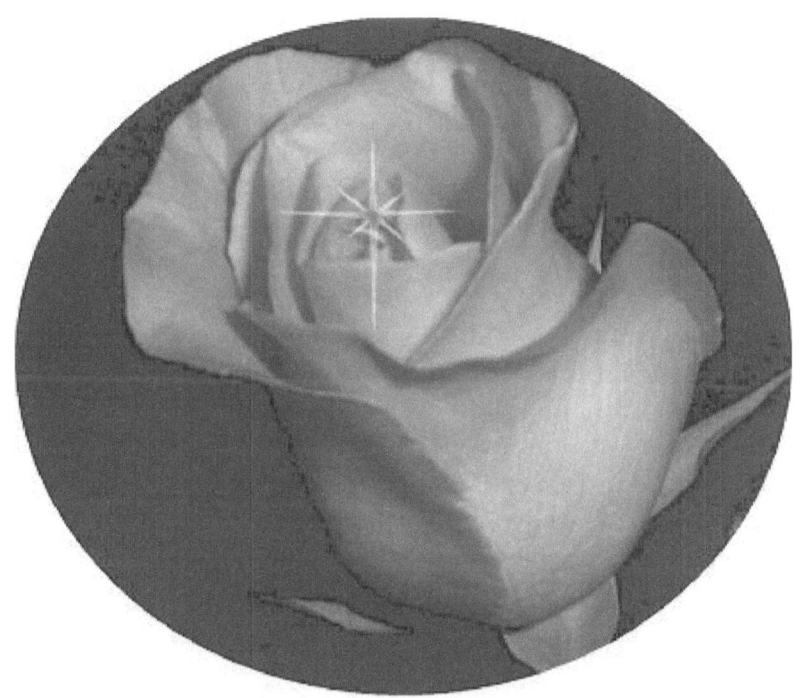

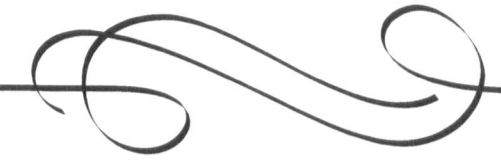

A PRAYER FOR YOU

I said a prayer for you today,
I hope you didn't mind.
I asked the Lord to comfort you
and put your tears behind.

I prayed for peace and mercy, too,
to help you through each day,
And for His loving guidance
as He leads you on your way.

You need not walk this path alone
so I prayed He'd hold your hand,
and offer you some guidance
in a way you'll understand.

I asked Him for little miracles
and to bless you every day.
Keep looking for the Rainbows -
and let Him light your way.

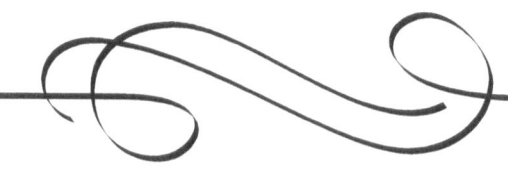

www.ingramcontent.com/pod-product-compliance
Lightning Source LLC
Chambersburg PA
CBHW052244290526
45785CB00016B/1279